Workbook

Essential
HEALTH

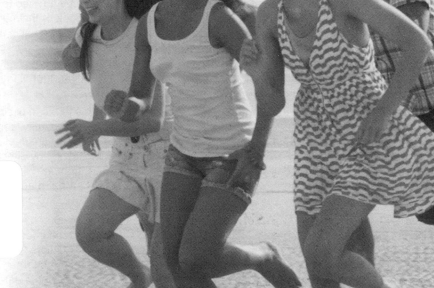

Publisher
The Goodheart-Willcox Company, Inc.
Tinley Park, Illinois
www.g-w.com

The Goodheart-Willcox Company, Inc. Brand Disclaimer: Brand names, company names, and illustrations for products and services included in this text are provided for educational purposes only and do not represent or imply endorsement or recommendation by the author or the publisher.

The Goodheart-Willcox Company, Inc. Safety Notice: The reader is expressly advised to carefully read, understand, and apply all safety precautions and warnings described in this book or that might also be indicated in undertaking the activities and exercises described herein to minimize risk of personal injury or injury to others. Common sense and good judgment should also be exercised and applied to help avoid all potential hazards. The reader should always refer to the appropriate manufacturer's technical information, directions, and recommendations; then proceed with care to follow specific equipment operating instructions. The reader should understand these notices and cautions are not exhaustive.

The publisher makes no warranty or representation whatsoever, either expressed or implied, including but not limited to equipment, procedures, and applications described or referred to herein, their quality, performance, merchantability, or fitness for a particular purpose. The publisher assumes no responsibility for any changes, errors, or omissions in this book. The publisher specifically disclaims any liability whatsoever, including any direct, indirect, incidental, consequential, special, or exemplary damages resulting, in whole or in part, from the reader's use or reliance upon the information, instructions, procedures, warnings, cautions, applications, or other matter contained in this book. The publisher assumes no responsibility for the activities of the reader.

The Goodheart-Willcox Company, Inc. Internet Disclaimer: The Internet resources and listings in this Goodheart-Willcox Publisher product are provided solely as a convenience to you. These resources and listings were reviewed at the time of publication to provide you with accurate, safe, and appropriate information. Goodheart-Willcox Publisher has no control over the referenced websites and, due to the dynamic nature of the Internet, is not responsible or liable for the content, products, or performance of links to other websites or resources. Goodheart-Willcox Publisher makes no representation, either expressed or implied, regarding the content of these websites, and such references do not constitute an endorsement or recommendation of the information or content presented. It is your responsibility to take all protective measures to guard against inappropriate content, viruses, or other destructive elements.

Cover Image: Monkey Business Images/Monkey Business/Thinkstock

Contents

Lesson 1.1

Key Terms Review

Multiple Choice: *Write the letter that corresponds to the correct answer in the blank space.*

_____ 1. Which of the following refers to a healthy balance of physical, emotional, intellectual, and social health?
   A. well-being
   B. optimal health
   C. wellness
   D. disorder

_____ 2. Which of the following does *not* describe a disorder?
   A. an abnormal physical condition
   B. a condition that appears to have no single cause
   C. a condition that has a single, specific, identified cause
   D. an abnormal mental condition

_____ 3. The flu and chicken pox are examples of _____.
   A. chronic diseases
   B. acute diseases
   C. disorders
   D. all of the above

_____ 4. Cancer, heart disease, and diabetes are examples of _____.
   A. chronic diseases
   B. acute diseases
   C. disorders
   D. all of the above

_____ 5. On the health and wellness continuum, the opposite of disease and early death is _____.
   A. chronic disease
   B. optimal health
   C. disorder
   D. acute disease

_____ 6. What traits characterize people who are in a state of well-being?
   A. They feel safe.
   B. They feel fulfilled.
   C. They feel productive.
   D. all of the above

_____ 7. A disease indicator that is sensed by the sick person is called a(n) _____.
   A. sign
   B. symptom
   C. impairment
   D. disorder

_____ 8. An outward indicator of disease that can be detected and measured by other people is a(n) _____.
   A. sign
   B. symptom
   C. impairment
   D. disorder

Matching: *Match each description with the name of the dimension of health it describes. Write the letter corresponding to the answer in the blank space. One term will not be used.*

_____ 9. involves communication skills, relationships, and the ability to interact with others

_____ 10. involves your body, including physical fitness and the ability to cope with everyday physical tasks

_____ 11. involves your emotions, mood, outlook on life, and beliefs about yourself

_____ 12. involves your ability to think clearly and critically, learn, and solve problems

A. emotional health

B. intellectual health

C. physical health

D. social health

E. optimal health

Lesson 1.1

The Four Dimensions of Health

The four dimensions of health—physical health, emotional health, intellectual health, and social health—are interrelated. A change in the state of one dimension often affects the other dimensions. In the boxes following each scenario, write the effects of the scenario on each dimension of the person's health.

1. Jermaine and his girlfriend split up. In the weeks following the breakup, Jermaine pulls away from his friends and his family. He spends hours alone in his room. He has problems sleeping through the night and often oversleeps. As a result, he regularly skips breakfast. He has trouble concentrating in class and does poorly on his midterm exams. To make things worse, he picks up a cold, followed by the flu.

Physical Health	Emotional Health
Intellectual Health	Social Health

2. Near the end of her senior year, Melanie is diagnosed with mononucleosis, a viral infection characterized by fatigue, sore throat, fever, and swollen lymph nodes. People with this illness can sometimes develop more serious medical problems. Melanie's doctor prescribes weeks of bed rest. Melanie can't go to school, play sports, appear in the school play, or attend some graduation parties she was looking forward to. The doctor says it may be several months before Melanie feels normal again. After several days, Melanie feels increasingly sad and upset and falls into depression.

Physical Health	Emotional Health
Intellectual Health	Social Health

3. Jeremy often feels jittery and unfocused. As a result, he has a hard time concentrating in class, and his teachers get annoyed with him. Jeremy has a hard time keeping up in class, which makes him feel bad about himself. Jeremy begins to drink alcohol in the attempt to cope with his negative feelings. After drinking one night, Jeremy is biking home when he runs a stop sign and gets knocked over by a car. He suffers a broken leg and collarbone.

Physical Health	Emotional Health
Intellectual Health	Social Health

Lesson 1.2

Finding Reliable Health Information

For this activity, you will find three sources of reliable information for each of the three topics listed below. You may use the sources of information given in Figure 1.6, "Health and Safety Information," or you may research your own sources. For each source, write the name of the organization and the title of the article or web page. If the source does not appear in Figure 1.6, list its website address as well. Do not use a source more than once.

Topic: *Shin splints*

1. A. Website #1 (name of organization) _____

   B. Title of article or web page _____

2. A. Website #2 (name of organization) _____

   B. Title of article or web page _____

3. A. Website #3 (name of organization) _____

   B. Title of article or web page _____

Topic: *Alcohol poisoning*

1. A. Website #1 (name of organization) _____

   B. Title of article or web page _____

2. A. Website #2 (name of organization) _____

   B. Title of article or web page _____

3. A. Website #3 (name of organization) _____

   B. Title of article or web page _____

Topic: *Acne*

1. A. Website #1 (name of organization) _____

   B. Title of article or web page _____

2. A. Website #2 (name of organization) _____

   B. Title of article or web page _____

3. A. Website #3 (name of organization) _____

   B. Title of article or web page _____

After compiling the above information about your sources, answer the following questions:

1. Of the three sources you chose for each topic, which sources were most reliable? How do you know?

_____

_____

2. Which sources provided the most interesting information? Write three facts you learned about each topic.

_____

_____

Lesson 1.2

Evaluating Health Information

Find an article that describes a research study and attach a copy of the article to this page. The article should describe a study that addresses a health and wellness topic; involves research on human subjects, not animals; and provides enough detail that you can answer the questions below.

1. What is the name of the publication or website in which the article appears? Does it qualify as a credible source? Why or why not?_____

   _____

2. Is information about the author(s) of the article given? If so, what is the name of the person or persons who wrote the article? What are the credentials and occupations of the author(s)?

   _____

   _____

3. Who conducted the research study, and what are the credentials of the researcher(s)? If little to no information about the researcher(s) is given, note that here._____

   _____

4. Does the article indicate the organization, government agency, institution, or business that funded, or paid for, the research? Does the funding organization benefit in some way from the research findings? If so, explain. _____

   _____

5. What was the sample size of the study? How many people participated as research subjects? A small sample size is problematic. _____

   _____

6. How were participants selected? Were they chosen randomly? Studies based on subjects who were not randomly chosen can sometimes be problematic.

   _____

   _____

7. Did the researchers use a control group in addition to the study group participants? A control group would be a group of people who were not exposed to the conditions of the research study. Studies conducted without control groups are usually not as rigorous as those that use control groups.

   _____

   _____

8. Summarize the conclusions of the study, including any recommendations or health advice given in the article. _____

   _____

   _____

9. Does the article inspire you to make changes to your lifestyle and choices? Explain.

   _____

   _____

Name _____ Date _____

Decision Making 101

Every day you make decisions that can affect your health and wellness. For example, you choose which foods to eat, how late you will stay up, who your friends are, and how you resolve conflicts with your parents or caregivers. Identify a health or wellness problem you are currently facing. Use the decision-making process to guide you in finding a solution and in putting the solution into action this week.

Step 1: Define the problem.

In the space below, briefly but accurately describe the problem you are facing.

_____

_____

_____

Step 2: Explore alternatives.

List three possible solutions to the problem and the pros (advantages) and cons (disadvantages) of each alternative. Your possible solutions should contain steps or actions that you can realistically begin to take this week.

Solution 1:

_____

Pros	Cons

Solution 2:

_____

Pros	Cons

(Continued)

Solution 3:

_____

Pros	Cons

Step 3: Select the best alternative.

Choose one of the solutions you listed. Which solution did you choose? Why?

_____

_____

_____

Step 4: Act on your decision.

Describe how you will act on your decision, and then take action. Afterward, explain how you acted on your decision and what happened or will happen as a result.

_____

_____

_____

_____

_____

_____

Step 5: Evaluate your decision.

Based on the consequences of your actions, do you think you made a good decision? Explain.

_____

_____

_____

_____

_____

_____

Name _____ Date _____

Goal Setting 101

In this activity, you will set a goal for improving your health this week. Your goal should be specific, and you should realistically be able to achieve it within one week. For example, an unrealistic goal might be, "I will lose thirty pounds this week." A realistic goal might be, "I will run outside for thirty minutes each evening this week." After recording a specific and realistic goal in the chart below, list specific steps you can take to reach that goal. If you are uncertain what steps you can take, confer with your teacher. Then, each day this week, check off the steps you took toward completing your goal. At the end of the week, analyze the results of your efforts by answering the questions at the bottom of the page.

Goal for Better Health							
Set a goal. Your goal should be *specific*, *realistic*, and *achievable*.							
Steps	Sun	Mon	Tues	Wed	Thurs	Fri	Sat

1. What circumstances, people, or resources were helpful as you tried to achieve your goal?

_____

_____

2. What circumstances, people, or resources hindered your progress or became obstacles to the achievement of your goal?

_____

_____

_____

3. Are you satisfied with the results of your efforts this week? Explain your answer.

_____

_____

_____

4. Do you need to revise your goal or the steps you will take to reach it? If so, explain how.

_____

_____

Name _____ Date _____

Communicating with Your Doctor

Communicating clearly and effectively with your healthcare providers is an important part of receiving good healthcare. In this exercise, you will partner with a classmate and act out a scene in which a patient visits his or her doctor about a health problem. One person in each pair will play the patient and the other will play the healthcare provider. Your classmates will evaluate how the patient communicates his or her problem and will suggest improvements.

As the Patient-Doctor Pair

Choose a health problem, such as a bad cold or a broken leg. On a separate sheet of paper or online, write a script in which a patient describes his or her problem to the doctor. The doctor can ask questions, if necessary, to obtain more information from the patient. You will act out this scene in front of the class.

As the Audience

While watching your classmates act out their scenes, answer the following questions for each pair.

1. Did the patient clearly describe his or her problem and symptoms? If not, what was unclear?

   _____

   _____

2. Were the patient's comments general or specific? If not, which points needed more detail?

   _____

   _____

3. Did the doctor have to ask follow-up questions to get more information?

   _____

   _____

4. Did the patient do a good job answering the doctor's questions? Why or why not?

   _____

   _____

5. Describe the body language of the patient and doctor during their interaction. What did the patient's body language convey?

   _____

   _____

6. Is there anything the patient could have done to improve the communication?

   _____

   _____

Chapter 1

Reading Practice

Reread the following passage from the textbook. Then answer the questions that follow.

A Continuum of Health

People often think of well-being as a dichotomy (one or the other)—you are either healthy or you are not. This is not, however, an accurate description of health. A person's health status normally lies somewhere between the extremes of poor and excellent. This range in health status is described as a *continuum*. Most people experience one or more problems that put their health status in the center of the wellness continuum.

Optimal health lies at one end of the continuum. Optimal health is not just the absence of disease. Optimal health is a state of superb health and wellness—excellent physical, emotional, intellectual, and social health. People want their health status to be at or near this end of the continuum.

At the other end of the continuum lies disease and premature death. The term *disease* describes an overall poor state of health in which people cannot function normally. As you'll learn, there are many types of diseases and disorders that can affect the body and the mind.

_____ 1. Based on the context, what is the definition of the word *dichotomy*?
- A. a range in health status
- B. a person's health status
- C. a division of two groups or entities that are mutually exclusive
- D. a state of superb health and wellness

_____ 2. Why is the range of health and wellness called a *continuum*?
- A. A person is either wholly healthy or wholly unhealthy.
- B. It is impossible to achieve optimal health and wellness.
- C. A person's health usually lies somewhere between premature death and optimal health and wellness.
- D. A person with optimal health and wellness will likely die prematurely.

_____ 3. Based on the context, what is the definition of the word *optimal*?
- A. least desirable
- B. most desirable
- C. neither most nor least desirable
- D. the absence of disease

_____ 4. The health status of most people lies at what point on the continuum of health and wellness?
- A. at disease and premature death
- B. at optimal health
- C. between optimal health and disease and premature death
- D. outside of the continuum

_____ 5. Which of the following statements about disease is *not* true?
- A. Disease is a state of health in which people cannot function normally.
- B. Disease describes an overall optimal state of health.
- C. Disease can affect the body and the mind.
- D. Disease describes an overall poor state of health.

_____ 6. What is the main idea of the passage?
- A. There are many types of diseases and disorders.
- B. People often think of well-being as a dichotomy.
- C. The health status of most people lies between the extremes of optimal and diseased.
- D. Optimal health is not just the absence of disease.

Chapter 1

Practice Test

Completion: *Write the term that completes the statement in the space provided.*

1. The ability to locate, interpret, and apply information pertaining to your health is called health _____.

2. _____ learning is the continuing pursuit of learning and studying throughout life.

3. A _____ is someone who purchases goods and services.

4. A 2010 law that expanded access to health insurance to more Americans and included a "Patient's Bill of Rights" was the _____.

5. The _____ division of the United States Department of Health and Human Services provides leadership, funding, and oversight of the healthcare system.

True/False: *Indicate whether each statement below is true or false by circling either T or F.*

T   F   6. A problem in one dimension of health will not affect other dimensions of health.

T   F   7. Reliable health information can usually be found on websites with URL stems of .gov, .edu, and .org.

T   F   8. The size or popularity of a newspaper or magazine is a good indicator of how much you can trust the information it provides.

T   F   9. Your actions can affect your health.

T   F   10. The healthcare field employs more people than any other type of business in the United States.

Multiple Choice: *Write the letter that corresponds to the correct answer in the blank space.*

_____ 11. Which of the following is true about the theories and health claims resulting from pseudoscience?
  A. They are based on experimentation and observation.
  B. They are peer-reviewed.
  C. They cannot be repeated.
  D. They are verified by other scientists.

_____ 12. The health claim, "Use this product for one week and get rid of acne forever!" is an example of _____.
  A. health promotion
  B. health literacy
  C. science
  D. pseudoscience

_____ 13. The _____ is a type of health insurance that only pays when the patient uses doctors and hospitals that are members of a network.
  A. primary care system
  B. health maintenance organization
  C. life and disability system
  D. preferred provider organization

_____ 14. A type of healthcare professional who can deliver primary care services, but who works under the supervision of physicians, is a(n) _____.
  A. osteopathic doctor
  B. specialist
  C. nurse
  D. physician assistant

_____ 15. _____ is a type of government-funded health insurance for people who are 65 years of age and older.
  A. The Affordable Care Act
  B. Medicare
  C. Medicaid
  D. Social Security

Name _____

Matching: *Match each medical or healthcare term to its definition by writing the letter of the term in the space provided.*

_____ 16. hospital where patients reside overnight

_____ 17. regular fee paid in exchange for insurance services

_____ 18. medical provider who is extensively training in one or two areas of health

_____ 19. recovery of function following surgery, disease, or injury

_____ 20. identification of a disease, disorder, or disability

_____ 21. use of medicine, surgery, counseling, or other therapy to deal with a condition

_____ 22. healthcare establishment where patients receive diagnoses and care, but do not stay overnight

_____ 23. doctor who provides routine checkups and screenings

_____ 24. services for reducing potential causes of diseases, disorders, and injuries

_____ 25. amount paid for healthcare services each year before a health insurance company begins to pay claims

A. deductible

B. diagnosis

C. generic drug

D. inpatient facility

E. outpatient facility

F. premium

G. prevention

H. primary care physician

I. rehabilitation

J. specialist

K. treatment

Analyzing Data: *Use the information provided to answer the following questions.*

Real-World Healthcare

The Tanakas are a family of four with two teenage children. They have a preferred provider organization (PPO) health insurance plan. Their monthly premium for the plan is $500. Their annual deductible is $2,000.

---

26. How much do the Tanakas spend on health insurance premiums each year?

_____

_____

27. Suppose 17-year-old Susan Tanaka breaks her leg while skateboarding. The doctor bills, emergency room visit, X-rays, prescription drugs, and other expenses add up to $700. It's early in the year and none of the family's deductible has been met. How much of the bill will be covered by the health insurance company? by the Tanakas?

_____

_____

28. Another plan is available to the Tanakas that charges a monthly premium of $350. The other plan is a health maintenance organization (HMO) plan. Over one year, how much money would the Tanakas save if they switched to the HMO plan? What would be a disadvantage of changing plans?

_____

_____

Short Answer: *On a separate piece of paper, answer the following questions using what you have learned in this chapter.*

29. Explain the difference between science and pseudoscience.

30. List three actions that consumers can take to lower their healthcare costs.

Lesson 2.1

Create a Quality of Life Index

One way to assess a person's health and wellness is to look at quality of life, or the person's satisfaction with various aspects of his or her life. You read about the Ferrans and Powers Quality of Life Index (QLI) which was developed by researchers to help measure a person's quality of life. Go to the University of Illinois at Chicago's website to view a generic version of the index. Then, create your own quality of life index for teenagers, based on what areas of satisfaction you think are most important. Ask a few classmates to fill it out.

Name _____

1. **Very Dissatisfied**
2. **Moderately Dissatisfied**
3. **Slightly Dissatisfied**
4. **Slightly Satisfied**
5. **Moderately Satisfied**
6. **Very Satisfied**

HOW *SATISFIED* ARE YOU WITH:						
Example: *The emotional support you get from your family?*	1	2	3	4	(5)	6
1.	1	2	3	4	5	6
2.	1	2	3	4	5	6
3.	1	2	3	4	5	6
4.	1	2	3	4	5	6
5.	1	2	3	4	5	6
6.	1	2	3	4	5	6
7.	1	2	3	4	5	6
8.	1	2	3	4	5	6
9.	1	2	3	4	5	6
10.	1	2	3	4	5	6
11.	1	2	3	4	5	6
12.	1	2	3	4	5	6

Name _____ Date _____

What Are the Risk Factors?

Risk factors are aspects of people's lives that increase the chances they will develop a disease or disorder, or experience an injury. Risk factors are categorized into three types: behavioral, environmental, and genetic. Risk factors can be either modifiable or non-modifiable. For each of the following scenarios, identify the teenager's risk factors for a disease, disorder, or injury. Identify types of risk factors by checking the appropriate boxes. Then suggest what each teenager can do to reduce or eliminate the risk factors.

1. Carlos is a 15-year-old who lives with his mother. When Carlos was 11 years old, his parents divorced, and his father moved away. Since then, Carlos has had frequent bouts of sadness and has had problems sleeping. His father and grandmother were diagnosed with depression.

   A. In the chart below, identify Carlos' risk factors for depression.

Risk Factor	Risk Factor Type			Modifiable or Non-modifiable?
	Behavioral	Environmental	Genetic	

   B. What steps can Carlos and his family take to reduce or eliminate these risk factors for depression?

   _____

2. Arianna lives in a neighborhood where gang members hang out and sell drugs. Shootings occur on a regular basis, usually caused by gang members targeting each other; but sometimes the shootings affect bystanders. When she is 15, Arianna begins to date a 17-year-old gang member, although her parents disapprove. She often sneaks out of her home late at night to meet him in the street.

   A. In the chart below, identify Arianna's risk factors for being a victim of gun violence.

Risk Factor	Risk Factor Type			Modifiable or Non-modifiable?
	Behavioral	Environmental	Genetic	

   B. What steps can Arianna, her family, and members of the community take to reduce or eliminate these risk factors?

   _____

How Safe Are You?

Read each of the following behaviors that impact your health and safety. Write the number that best describes your safety practices in the space provided. Then total your score. The higher your score, the safer you are.

1—Never

2—Once in a while

3—Sometimes

4—Most of the time

5—Always

_____ 1. I wear a helmet when bicycling.

_____ 2. I wear a seat belt when riding in a car.

_____ 3. I get more than one hour of physical activity a day.

_____ 4. I get at least nine hours of sleep a night.

_____ 5. I avoid foods that are high in calories, fat, or salt.

_____ 6. I do not smoke cigarettes.

_____ 7. I do not ride with someone who texts while driving.

_____ 8. I do not ride with drivers who have been drinking alcohol.

_____ 9. I do not ride in cars with others who are under 18 years of age.

_____ 10. I avoid being outdoors during thunderstorms or other severe weather situations.

_____ **Total score**

Name _____   Date _____

Making Healthy Decisions

Behavioral (lifestyle) risk factors are choices and behaviors that increase a person's chances of developing a disease, unhealthy condition, or injury. Almost everyone has behavioral risk factors that they can reduce or eliminate. For example, some people are physically inactive; others drink alcohol or smoke. Many people don't get enough sleep or spend time in tanning beds. For this activity, identify a behavioral risk factor that you want to change. Complete this exercise to determine how you can reduce or eliminate the risk factor.

1. Describe a behavioral risk factor that may put your health at risk, now or in the future.

   _____

2. Brainstorm and then list three specific actions you could take to eliminate or reduce the risk factor.

   A. _____

   B. _____

   C. _____

3. In the tables below, identify the pros and cons for each action.

A.

Pros	Cons

B.

Pros	Cons

C.

Pros	Cons

4. Which action will most effectively reduce or eliminate your risk factor? Please explain.

   _____

   _____

Name _____ Date _____

What Do You Know about Genes?

Matching: *Match each of the terms below with one of the statements by writing the letter of the term in the space provided.*

_____ 1. contains the blueprint for the structure and function of your cells; directs how you grow and develop

_____ 2. a specialized compartment of a cell that holds genetic material

_____ 3. package of genes that are bundled together; you inherit a set from each parent

_____ 4. the chemical of which genes are composed

_____ 5. unit that makes up the tissues of the body

A. cell

B. chromosome

C. deoxyribonucleic acid (DNA)

D. gene

E. nucleus

Matching: *Match the following words with the structures they describe.*

A. nucleus

B. chromosome

C. gene

D. DNA

E. cell

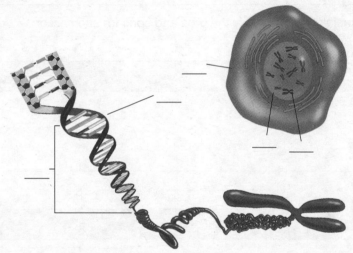

Courtesy of the National Institute of General Medical Sciences

Identify: *Identify whether each of the following health problems have genetic risk factors that are passed down from one generation to another.*

Disease or Disorder	Genetic Risk Factor	No Genetic Risk Factor
common cold		
diabetes		
broken arm		
sickle cell anemia		
heart disease		
depression		
skin cancer		
drug overdose		
colon cancer		

Name _____ Date _____

Reducing Genetic Risk Factors

Genetic risk factors for diseases and disorders are generally non-modifiable. However, many diseases and disorders are caused by the interplay of behavioral and environmental risk factors with genetic risk factors. If a disease runs in your family, you can often make changes to your behavior and environment to reduce the chance you will develop the disease. For each of the following scenarios, identify each person's risk factors and describe what the person can do to avoid developing a disease or disorder.

1. Type 2 diabetes mellitus runs in Jonelle's family. Jonelle's mother developed it when she was in her 50s. Jonelle, who is 16, is overweight and gets very little physical activity, except for the occasional walk to school. She usually gets a ride to school. Also, the kitchen cupboards and refrigerator in her home are always stocked with high-calorie foods.

   A. List Jonelle's genetic, behavioral, and environmental risk factors for type 2 diabetes mellitus.

   _____

   _____

   B. What can she do to lower or eliminate this risk?

   _____

   _____

2. Last summer before his senior year, Thomas worked as a lifeguard and noticed the extra attention he got because of his bronzed skin. After summer ended, Thomas visited a nearby tanning parlor regularly and lay in a tanning bed. His father recently had to have a patch of skin removed because he had developed skin cancer. But Thomas isn't worried. None of his friends wear sunscreen, and they don't worry about skin cancer.

   A. List Thomas' genetic, behavioral, and environmental risk factors for skin cancer.

   _____

   _____

   B. What can he do to lower or eliminate this risk?

   _____

   _____

3. Colon cancer took the life of Josh's uncle when he was only 45. Josh's uncle was overweight, physically inactive, a heavy drinker, and a smoker. When Josh's uncle was alive, Josh hung out at his house where they played video games for hours. Although he broke the law, Josh's uncle gave Josh beer and cigarettes. Josh, who is 15, continues to smoke and drink, and does not exercise.

   A. List Josh's genetic, behavioral, and environmental risk factors for colon cancer.

   _____

   _____

   B. What can he do to lower or eliminate this risk?

   _____

   _____

Lesson 2.4

Who Is Most at Risk?

Read each pair of descriptions and place an R in the blank beside the person who has the greater amount of environmental or socioeconomic risk factors. You may have to do some research. Explain why you made the choice you did and cite one or more facts.

1. _____college graduate   _____high school graduate

   Why? _____

2. _____firefighter   _____website designer

   Why? _____

3. _____resident of humid climate   _____resident of temperate climate

   Why? _____

4. _____high-income earner   _____low-income earner

   Why? _____

5. _____someone who lives next to a forest _____someone who lives next to a highway

   Why? _____

6. _____power tool operator   _____surgeon

   Why? _____

7. _____restaurant cook   _____waiter or waitress

   Why? _____

8. _____X-ray technician   _____dental hygienist

   Why? _____

9. _____librarian   _____farm worker

   Why? _____

10. _____bookkeeper   _____taxi driver

    Why? _____

Lesson 2.4

Environmental Hazards

It is important to know where you can go for information about the various hazards present in your current or future environments. In this activity, you will track down a few reliable agencies and organizations, and you will summarize what environmental hazards you learn about.

1. Centers for Disease Control and Prevention

   A. What is this agency's website address?

   _____

   B. What is the agency's mission, or how does the agency describe itself?

   _____

   C. Give three examples of environmental hazards the agency is concerned with.

   _____

   _____

2. National Weather Service

   A. What is this agency's website address?

   _____

   B. What is the agency's mission, or how does the agency describe itself?

   _____

   C. Give three examples of environmental hazards the agency is concerned with.

   _____

   _____

3. Your State Government

   A. What is the name and website address of your state's health or public health department?

   _____

   B. What is the agency's mission, or how does the agency describe itself?

   _____

   C. Give three examples of environmental hazards the agency is concerned with.

   _____

   _____

4. World Health Organization

   A. What is this agency's website address?

   _____

   B. What is the organization's mission, or how does it describe itself?

   _____

   C. Give three examples of environmental hazards the agency is concerned with.

   _____

   _____

Chapter 2

Reading Practice

Reread the following passage from the textbook. Then answer the questions that follow.

Physical Activity in the Workplace

Some types of work require regular and sometimes vigorous activity, while other jobs entail almost no physical activity. Studies of different occupations have found considerable differences in physical activity.

The level of physical activity is reflected in the number of *calories*—units of energy—used to perform that activity. For example, compare the physical activity levels of three average men who weigh 155 pounds. The first man, a website designer, works mainly at a desk and uses about 102 calories per hour. The second man, a carpenter, uses about 260 calories each hour as he lifts heavy objects and runs errands. The third man, a firefighter, carries a heavy pack and works in extreme conditions. He uses about 892 calories per hour.

What if these three men never exercised outside of the workplace? In particular, if the website designer does not get regular physical activity outside of work, he leads a sedentary, inactive lifestyle. This type of lifestyle can lead to weight gain and cardiovascular disease.

The total amount of physical activity in your day affects your health. That is why it is important for students to get physical activity outside of school, where they spend most of their time sitting. People whose work requires them to be inactive most of the day should also plan physical activity outside of work. Your level of activity at school or work is not a modifiable risk factor, but you control your level of physical activity at home. Simple changes such as waking up early to jog, walk, or bike can increase your level of physical activity and improve your health.

_____ 1. Based on the context, what is the definition of the word *vigorous*?

  A. physical activity that uses little energy

  B. physical activity that uses much energy

  C. physical activity performed while seated

  D. physical activity performed while standing

_____ 2. Which of the following is a sedentary activity?

  A. watching television

  B. playing basketball

  C. walking to school

  D. vacuuming a carpet

_____ 3. Which occupation involves the lowest level of physical activity?

  A. textbook writer

  B. firefighter

  C. carpenter

  D. physical education teacher

_____ 4. What is the main idea of the passage?

  A. Website designers are less healthy than firefighters and carpenters.

  B. To avoid health problems, people with sedentary jobs should be more physically active.

  C. Your level of activity at school or work is not a modifiable risk factor.

  D. Studies of different occupations have found considerable differences in physical activity.

Chapter 2

Practice Test

Completion: *Write the term that completes the statement in the space provided.*

1. The average life expectancy for all Americans has _____ significantly in 50 years.

2. Compared with a person who does not have a risk factor for a disease, the person with a risk factor has a _____ chance of developing the disease.

3. Type 2 diabetes mellitus is a disorder resulting in a _____ blood sugar level.

4. Infectious diseases are caused by microscopic living things called _____.

5. Texting while driving is an example of _____ driving behavior.

True/False: *Indicate whether each statement below is true or false by circling either T or F.*

T   F   6. The more risk factors for a particular disease a person has, the greater the chance he or she will develop the disease.

T   F   7. A person who appears to be doing well can have a poor quality of life.

T   F   8. Accidents happen to people and cannot be prevented.

T   F   9. More than half of drivers who are 16–24 years of age do not use seat belts.

T   F 10. College graduates are less likely to be overweight or obese than people who are less educated.

Multiple Choice: *Write the letter that corresponds to the correct answer in the blank space.*

_____ 11. Which of the following is *not* an environmental risk factor?
    A. climate
    B. workplace
    C. behavior
    D. geography

_____ 12. The main cause of skin cancer is _____.
    A. genes
    B. exposure to ultraviolet radiation
    C. diet
    D. none of the above

_____ 13. Colon cancer is caused by _____.
    A. genes
    B. lifestyle factors
    C. behavioral factors
    D. all of the above

_____ 14. Which type of risk factor is non-modifiable?
    A. genetic risk factors
    B. behavioral risk factors
    C. environmental risk factors
    D. all of the above

_____ 15. Heart disease and cancer combined cause nearly _____% of all deaths in the United States.
    A. 10
    B. 25
    C. 50
    D. 75

(Continued)

Matching: *Match each term to its definition by writing the letter of the term in the space provided.*

_____ 16. person's level of satisfaction with various aspects of his or her life

_____ 17. factors that involve a person's level of education, type of work, income level, and access to healthcare

_____ 18. choices and behaviors that increase your chance of developing a disease, unhealthy condition, or injury

_____ 19. actual number of years a person lives

_____ 20. number of deaths caused by a disease, disorder, injury, or other condition in a population

_____ 21. estimate of how long a person is likely to live

_____ 22. characteristics of your surroundings that may cause you injury or illness

A. behavioral risk factors

B. environmental risk factors

C. inherited disease

D. life expectancy

E. life span

F. mortality

G. quality of life

H. socioeconomic risk factors

Analyzing Data: *Use the information provided to answer the following questions.*

Life Expectancy at Birth, 1970 and 2001 (or nearest year)

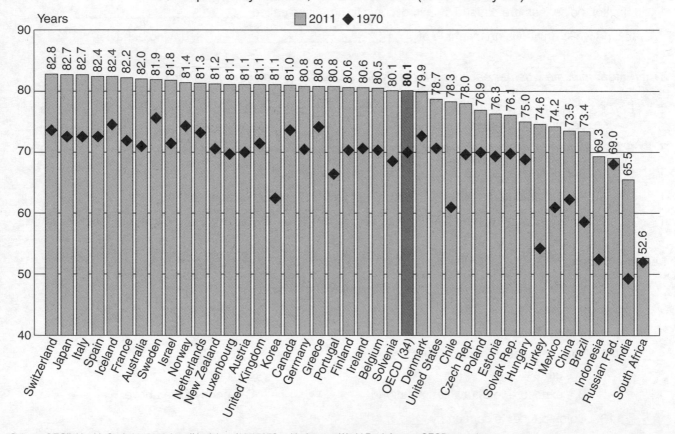

Source: OECD Health Statistics 2013, http://dx.doi.org/10.1787/health-data-en; World Bank for non-OECD countries.

23. The column labeled *OECD (34)* gives the life expectancy in years for all thirty-four OECD (Organization for Economic Cooperation and Development) member countries. What was the life expectancy at birth for the OECD member countries in 2011?

_____

24. What was the life expectancy of people in the United States in 2011, and how does it compare with the life expectancy for all OECD member countries that year?

_____

Short Answer: *On a separate sheet of paper, answer the following questions using what you have learned in this chapter.*

25. Contrast modifiable risk factors and non-modifiable risk factors. Give two examples of each.

26. Explain why life expectancy and life span can be different due to behavioral risk factors.

Lesson 3.1

Key Terms Review

Multiple Choice: *Write the letter that corresponds to the correct answer in the blank space.*

_____ 1. Which nutrient provides the body with quick energy?
     A. proteins   C. carbohydrates
     B. vitamins   D. fats

_____ 2. Sugar, starch, and fiber belong to which family of nutrients?
     A. proteins   C. carbohydrates
     B. minerals   D. fats

_____ 3. Which food is a complex carbohydrate?
     A. table sugar   C. water
     B. beans   D. oil

_____ 4. Which food is a simple carbohydrate?
     A. table sugar   C. water
     B. beans   D. oil

_____ 5. Which nutrient is *not* a source of energy for the body?
     A. proteins   C. carbohydrates
     B. fiber   D. fats

_____ 6. Which nutrient is used to build and maintain all of the cells and tissues in the body?
     A. proteins   C. fats
     B. carbohydrates   D. water

_____ 7. Which nutrient provides more calories per gram than any other nutrient?
     A. proteins   C. fats
     B. carbohydrates   D. minerals

_____ 8. _____ are chemical units that join to make proteins.
     A. Fatty acids   C. Hormones
     B. Glucose molecules   D. Amino acids

_____ 9. In which form is energy for the body stored in the muscles and liver?
     A. glycogen   C. sucrose
     B. glucose   D. amino acids

_____ 10. When people do not have enough calcium in their diets during childhood and adolescence, they raise their risk for developing _____.
     A. anemia   C. dehydration
     B. osteoporosis   D. cretinism

Matching: *Match each statement about fats to the type of fat it describes by writing the appropriate letter in the blank space. Answers may be used more than once.*

_____ 11. solid at room temperature and found primarily in animal-based foods   A. saturated fat

_____ 12. found in animal-based foods and also made by the body   B. trans fat

_____ 13. most dangerous type of fat and found in many processed foods   C. unsaturated fat

_____ 14. liquid at room temperature   D. cholesterol

Lesson 3.1

Vitamin and Mineral Review

Use figures 3.6 and 3.7 of the student text to answer the following questions about vitamins and minerals.

1. A. Which vitamins and minerals are necessary for building strong, healthy bones?

   _____

   _____

   B. List five foods you can eat to build strong, healthy bones.

   _____

   _____

   _____

   _____

   _____

2. A. Which vitamin maintains the health of the retina, which is important for good eyesight?

   _____

   B. List five foods that contain this vitamin.

   _____

   _____

   _____

   _____

   _____

3. A. Which vitamin or mineral carries oxygen from the lungs to the rest of the body?

   _____

   B. List three sources of this vitamin or mineral.

   _____

   _____

   _____

4. A. Which minerals help regulate the body's fluid balance?

   _____

   _____

   B. List three sources of these minerals.

   _____

   _____

   _____

Name _____

5. A. Which vitamin promotes healing and is essential for healthy teeth and gums?

_____

   B. List three sources of this vitamin.

_____

_____

_____

6. A. Which vitamin is essential to cell division and the growth and production of healthy red blood cells?

_____

   B. List three sources of this vitamin.

_____

_____

_____

7. A. Which vitamin is important for blood coagulation and blood clotting?

_____

   B. List three sources of this vitamin.

_____

_____

_____

8. A. Which mineral assists with the production of thyroid hormones?

_____

   B. List three sources of this mineral.

_____

_____

_____

9. A. Which vitamins are fat-soluble?

_____

   B. Explain how fat-soluble vitamins are different from water-soluble vitamins.

_____

_____

10. A. What are the two types of minerals?

_____

_____

   B. Explain the difference between the two types.

_____

_____

_____

Name _____ Date _____

Evaluate Your Diet

The first step to eating more healthfully is to become aware of what you are eating now. In this four-part activity, you will compare what you are eating now to what is recommended by the Dietary Guidelines for Americans.

Part 1: Complete a Three-Day Food Log

In a notebook or online, record everything you eat and drink for three days. This includes meals, snacks, and water and other beverages. Estimate the serving size for every food or beverage you consume. You can base your estimations on the sample serving size chart provided below.

Sample Serving Sizes (1 serving)				
Grains Group	**Protein Foods Group**	**Fruit Group**	**Vegetable Group**	**Dairy Group**
1 slice bread 1 cup cereal ½ cup cooked pasta or rice	1 egg 1 Tbsp. peanut butter ½ ounce nuts 1 ounce of lean meat, poultry, or fish	1 cup raw or cooked 1 cup fruit juice 1 medium piece of fruit	1 cup raw or cooked 2 cups raw leafy 1 cup vegetable juice	1 cup milk 1 cup yogurt 1½ ounces cheese

Part 2: Sort Foods into Food Groups

Review your food log from the past three days, and assign each item in your log to one or more food groups.

	Grains	Protein Foods	Fruit	Vegetables	Dairy
Day 1					
Day 2					
Day 3					
Total Servings					

Name _____

Part 3: Research Recommended Amounts

For each food group, calculate the average number of servings you ate and enter the numbers into the second column of the chart below. (To calculate the average, add up all of the servings you ate in a food group for the three days and divide by three.)

Next, go to ChooseMyPlate.gov and calculate your daily food plan. Answer the questions about your age, gender, height, weight, and activity level. The daily food plan will give you the recommended amounts of each food group you should eat to stay healthy. Write those amounts in the third column of the chart. Then subtract the number in the second column from the number in the third column and enter that number in the fourth column.

Food Group	Amount You Had (Average of 3 days)	Recommended Amount	Subtract Amount You Had from Recommended Amount
Grains			
Protein			
Fruit			
Vegetables			
Dairy			

Part 4: Drawing Conclusions

Review the results of your calculations from part 3, and then answer the following questions:

1. Did you eat more than the recommended amount in any food group? Which group(s)?

   _____

   _____

2. Did you eat less than the recommended amount in any food group? Which group(s)?

   _____

   _____

Lesson 3.2

Calculating Calories

Four meals are illustrated in Figure 3.9 of your textbook: a fried chicken and fries meal and three healthier options. Fill in the blanks in the chart below to calculate how many calories are contained in each meal; some of the values are filled in for you. Go to the website of the United States Department of Agriculture (USDA). Look up food values in the USDA's databases (Nutritive Value of Foods and National Nutrient Database for Standard Reference). These databases list calories, fat grams, and nutrients contained in many types of foods and drinks. Remember to calculate calories and total fat for the serving sizes given below. Then answer the questions that follow.

Original Meal	Calories	Total Fat (grams)
3 drumsticks of fried chicken	____	____
medium-size serving of fries (fried in oil)	____	____
Total calories	____	____
Healthy Option 1		
Whole-wheat turkey wrap		
1 whole-wheat tortilla	127	4.0
2 slices deli turkey breast	64	0.5
¼ cup raw vegetables	5	0
2 tsp. fat-free mustard	____	0
1 apple, sliced	____	0
Total calories	____	____
Healthy Option 2		
Grilled chicken salad		
2 cups lettuce	____	0
3-oz. skinless, grilled chicken breast	102	2.2
½ cup bread croutons	58	1.0
1 Tbsp. olive oil for grilling	____	____
1 Tbsp. low-fat mayonnaise	49	5.0
Total calories	____	____
Healthy Option 3		
1 skinless, grilled chicken breast	____	____
1 cup roasted sweet potatoes in 2 tsp. oil	122	5.0
1 cup raw vegetables	8	0
2 Tbsp. low-fat salad dressing (Italian)	____	____
Total calories	____	____

Name _____ Date _____

Analyzing Data: *Answer the following questions based on your findings.*

1. Which meal contains the most calories? the least?

    _____

    _____

    _____

    _____

2. Which meal contains the most grams of fat? the least?

    _____

    _____

    _____

    _____

3. Which foods contain the least amount of fat?

    _____

    _____

    _____

    _____

4. How are fat and calories related?

    _____

    _____

    _____

    _____

Lesson 3.3

Decision Making at the Grocery Store

Luke goes grocery shopping for his family. He wants to fill his cart with nutritious foods and avoid items that are less healthful—or contain excess sugar, fats, and empty calories. In this activity, you will answer questions for Luke as he shops at the grocery store.

1. Luke pauses in front of the dairy case, ready to grab a carton of milk. His choices are: whole milk, low-fat milk, and fat-free milk. Which carton should he put into his cart? Explain your answer.

   _____

   _____

   _____

2. In the bread aisle, Luke spots a loaf of bread in a colorful wrapper that reads "Made with Whole Grains." However, the list of ingredients begins with: enriched flour, water, whole-wheat flour. Should Luke buy the bread?

   _____

   _____

   _____

3. In the freezer aisle, Luke looks for an ice cream that is low in fat and calories. The Nutrition Facts label for Product A lists 300 calories per serving, which looks good compared to Product B which lists 500 calories per serving. The serving size listed on the Nutrition Facts label is ½ cup for Product A and 1 cup for Product B. Which ice cream has fewer calories?

   _____

   _____

   _____

4. For an energy pick-me-up, Luke likes to snack on an "energy" bar in the afternoon between classes. He is looking for a product that contains the most protein per serving. Where on the Nutrition Facts labels should Luke look to determine which energy bars have the most protein?

   _____

   _____

   _____

5. Luke swings by the juice aisle to buy some apple juice for his 3-year-old sister. His mother told him to choose a brand that has little added sugar. He finds a product that does not list sugar. The ingredients list reads: filtered water, high-fructose corn syrup, corn syrup, apple juice from concentrate. Should he buy this product?

   _____

   _____

   _____

Lesson 3.3

Eat It or Toss It?

Read each of the following food-safety scenarios and determine whether the food in question should be eaten or thrown away. Identify any food-safety hazards in the scenarios and explain how the hazards can be fixed or avoided.

1. Deidre is making hamburgers for her family for dinner. She prepares half a dozen hamburger patties and puts them into a pan on the stove. After a short time, the patties are brown on the outside, although when she pokes one with a fork, red juice runs out. She decides the burgers are ready and takes them off the stove.

   A. Should Deidre eat or toss the hamburgers? Explain.

   _____

   B. What should Deidre do differently?

   _____

2. Xavier is preparing to cook chicken on his outdoor grill. He removes the pieces of raw chicken from the store wrapper and places them on a cutting board. He seasons the chicken and puts the pieces on the grill. While the chicken is cooking, Xavier makes a salad. Using the same cutting board, he cuts up vegetables for the salad.

   A. Should Xavier eat or toss the salad? Explain.

   _____

   B. What should Xavier do differently?

   _____

3. It's Amanda's job to clean up after dinner. One night, she postpones cleaning up because some friends stop by and they go to a movie. Four hours later, Amanda returns to the kitchen where the uneaten food is still in serving dishes on the counter. She covers the dishes and puts the food into the refrigerator so she and her family can eat the leftovers tomorrow.

   A. Should Amanda eat or toss the leftovers? Explain.

   _____

   B. What should Amanda do differently?

   _____

4. While babysitting his 2-year-old nephew, Jaden, Jerome stops at a fast-food restaurant for a snack. After ordering, Jerome watches while Jaden plays in the play structure with other small children. After a few minutes, Jaden returns to the table, pours a bunch of fries onto the table, and begins to eat them with his hands.

   A. Should Jerome and Jaden eat or toss the fries? Explain.

   _____

   B. What should Jerome and Jaden do differently?

   _____

5. Janessa stops by her friend Jamila's home to see how she is feeling. Earlier in the day, Jamila complained of feeling feverish and sick to her stomach. Jamila tells Janessa that she still feels ill; however, she has baked a batch of cookies. She picks up and passes Janessa a cookie to take home.

   A. Should Janessa eat or toss the cookie? Explain.

   _____

   B. What should Jamila do differently?

   _____

Chapter 3

Reading Practice

Reread the following passage from the textbook. Then answer the questions that follow.

As you learned earlier in this chapter, nutrients provide the body with the energy it needs to function. The energy provided by food is measured in terms of a unit called a *calorie*. Foods that provide larger amounts of energy are higher in calories than foods that provide smaller amounts of energy.

Some types of nutrients provide more calories than others. Carbohydrates and protein each provide 4 calories per gram. Fats provide 9 calories per gram, more than any other source.

Your calorie balance in a given day is determined by two distinct factors:

- the number of calories you consume through eating and drinking (this is energy *in* to your body)
- the number of calories you burn through the work of your *metabolism* and your daily physical activities (this is energy *out* of your body)

Your body burns calories to perform the many functions of your metabolism that keep you alive, such as eating, sleeping, and breathing. You also burn calories in the course of daily life—while walking to class, lifting a heavy backpack, and cleaning your room.

Maintaining Weight

You can maintain your weight by balancing calories consumed with calories burned throughout the day.

Calories in = Calories burned

Gaining Weight

When you consume more calories than your body burns, an energy imbalance occurs. The number of calories you take in and burn doesn't have to balance each day. If you take in more calories than you burn over time, however, you will gain weight. Those extra calories are stored in the body (mostly as fat).

Calories in > Calories burned

Losing Weight

An energy imbalance also occurs if, over time, you burn more calories than you take in. As you can probably guess, if you burn more than you consume, you will lose weight.

Calories in < Calories burned

_____ 1. Which concept does the author assume you understand before reading this passage?
- A. A unit called a calorie is used to measure the amount of energy provided by food.
- B. High-calorie foods provide more energy than low-calorie foods.
- C. Nutrients provide the body with energy.
- D. Metabolism includes functions that keep you alive.

_____ 2. Which of the following supports the statement that some nutrients provide more calories than others?
- A. The energy provided by food is measured in terms of a unit called a calorie.
- B. Foods that provide larger amounts of energy are higher in calories than foods that provide smaller amounts of energy.
- C. Carbohydrates and protein each provide 4 calories per gram. Fats provide 9 calories per gram.
- D. When you consume more calories than your body burns, an energy imbalance occurs.

_____ 3. What will happen if you regularly consume more calories than your body burns?
   A. You will gain weight.
   B. You will lose weight.
   C. Your weight will stay the same.
   D. You will have less energy.

_____ 4. If someone wants to lose weight, what must he or she do?
   A. burn more calories and consume more calories
   B. burn as many calories as he or she takes in
   C. burn fewer calories than he or she takes in
   D. burn more calories than he or she takes in

_____ 5. Which of the following is *not* a factor that determines your calorie balance?
   A. the number of calories you consume through eating and drinking
   B. the number of calories you planned on consuming
   C. the number of calories you burn through the work of your metabolism
   D. the number of calories you burn performing your daily physical activities

_____ 6. Which of the following playground images is helpful in understanding the author's description of energy?
   A. monkey bars
   B. a teeter-totter
   C. a slide
   D. a swing

_____ 7. What main idea concludes this passage?
   A. Your body weight is determined over time by how many calories you take in and how many calories you burn.
   B. Your body needs calories during activities such as walking to class, lifting a heavy backpack, and cleaning your room.
   C. Your body turns calories into energy for physical activity.
   D. Fats provide twice as many calories as carbohydrates or protein.

Chapter 3

Practice Test

Completion: *Write the term that completes the statement in the space provided.*

1. The three types of nutrients that provide energy to your body are carbohydrates, fat, and _____.

2. The body obtains energy by breaking down carbohydrates into _____.

3. _____ is a dangerous condition in which the body loses more fluids than it takes in.

4. A _____ food is a food that has relatively few calories but is rich in vitamins, minerals, and other substances that positively affect your health.

5. Substances that are added to food products to extend the products' shelf lives or improve their flavors are called food _____.

True/False: *Indicate whether each statement below is true or false by circling either T or F.*

T F 6. People should avoid eating any fats, if possible.

T F 7. Saturated fats are found primarily in animal-based foods and are solid at room temperature.

T F 8. Overnutrition occurs when people consume more calories than they need.

T F 9. In a food label's ingredients list, ingredients are listed by how nutritious they are.

T F 10. The government agency that regulates the labeling of food products is the United States Department of Agriculture (USDA).

Multiple Choice: *Write the letter that corresponds to the correct answer in the blank space.*

_____ 11. Sugars that occur naturally in some foods, including fruit, maple syrup, and dairy products, are _____.

    A. complex carbohydrates   C. glycogen

    B. simple carbohydrates   D. cholesterol

_____ 12. Your body only requires very small amounts of this type of nutrient to function properly.

    A. carbohydrates   C. proteins

    B. water   D. vitamins

_____ 13. _____ is a tough complex carbohydrate that the body is unable to digest.

    A. Fiber   C. Fructose

    B. Sugar   D. Sucrose

_____ 14. The energy provided by food is measured in a unit called a _____.

    A. pound   C. degree

    B. calorie   D. gram

_____ 15. _____ is a graphic designed to remind people about how much of each food group they should eat at a meal.

    A. The *Dietary Guidelines for Americans*   C. A Nutrition Facts label

    B. Daily Values   D. MyPlate

Name _____

Matching: *Match each key term to its definition by writing the letter of the term in the space provided.*

_____ 16. rate at which the body uses energy

_____ 17. description of food that is produced without chemical pesticides, bioengineering, or high-energy radiation

_____ 18. illness caused by toxins an organism has produced in a food

_____ 19. condition, characterized by weakness, fatigue, and headaches; occurs when people do not ingest enough iron

_____ 20. chemical units that make up proteins

_____ 21. chemical messengers that influence the basic processes in your body

_____ 22. type of fat that is made by the body and is also present in some foods

A. amino acids

B. anemia

C. cholesterol

D. foodborne intoxication

E. hormones

F. metabolism

G. organic

Analyzing Data: *Use the Nutrition Facts labels provided to answer the following questions.*

Tortilla Chips

Nutrition Facts
Serving Size 1 oz. (28g/About 6 chips)
Servings Per Container 9

Amount Per Serving

Calories 130   Calories from Fat 50

	% Daily Value*
Total Fat 6g	9%
Saturated Fat 1g	9%
Trans Fat 0g	
Cholesterol 0mg	0%
Sodium 80mg	3%
Total Carbohydrate 19g	6%
Dietary Fiber 1g	5%
Sugars 0g	
Protein 2g	
Vitamin A 0%	Vitamin C 0%
Calcium 4%	Iron 0%

Snack Mix

Nutrition Facts
Serving Size ¼ cup (32g)
Servings Per Container 6

Amount Per Serving

Calories 170   Calories from Fat 90

	% Daily Value*
Total Fat 11g	17%
Saturated Fat 3g	15%
Trans Fat 0g	
Polyunsaturated Fat 4g	
Monosaturated Fat 4g	
Cholesterol 0mg	0%
Sodium 80mg	5%
Potassiuum 115mg	3%
Total Carbohydrate 14g	5%
Dietary Fiber 2g	6%
Sugars 8g	
Protein 4g	
Vitamin A 0%	Vitamin C 2%
Calcium 2%	Iron 4%

23. Which food contains the fewest calories per serving?

_____

24. Which food contains the most calories from fat per serving?

_____

25. The Nutrition Facts label for snack mix lists four types of fats. What are the differences between trans fats and saturated fats? What impacts can they have on the body?

_____

_____

_____

Short Answer: *On a separate sheet of paper, answer the following questions using what you have learned in this chapter.*

26. Explain the concept of *calorie balance* and how it can be maintained. What happens when calorie balance is not maintained?

27. Compare and contrast food allergy and food intolerance.

Lesson 4.1

Problems with Comparisons

Teenagers who experience changes in weight and body composition may sometimes conclude that they are overweight. However, as you have learned in this chapter, weight and body composition are not always so straightforward. For each of the following scenarios, read carefully and answer the questions.

1. Stephanie and Mary are both 16. They are the same height, but Stephanie weighs 15 more pounds than Mary. Stephanie concludes that she is overweight. Is she correct? Are there any factors she may not be considering? Explain your answer.

   _____

   _____

   _____

   _____

2. Janet finds out that her body-fat percentage is 25%. Her boyfriend, Lucas, has a body-fat percentage of 15%. Janet believes that she is overweight because her body-fat percentage is higher than her boyfriend's. Is Janet correct? Are there any factors she may not be considering? Explain your answer.

   _____

   _____

   _____

   _____

3. In the ninth grade, Trevor and Louis are both 5 feet 8 inches tall and they have the same weight. But by the end of the tenth grade, Trevor has grown 2 inches, while Louis has grown 5 inches. What would you expect about Louis' weight in comparison with Trevor's weight by the end of the tenth grade?

   _____

   _____

   _____

   _____

4. Kris and Nancy have been best friends since elementary school. In elementary school, they wore the same size of clothing and often shared and swapped clothes. By the beginning of seventh grade, however, Kris can no longer fit into Nancy's smaller-sized clothing because her hips have grown wider. Kris concludes that she is overweight. Is Kris correct? Are there any factors she may not be considering? Explain.

   _____

   _____

   _____

   _____

5. Lawrence and Diego, both 17 years old, are cousins. Diego is a member of the school swim team and works out regularly. Lawrence leads a sedentary lifestyle and does not exercise much. Diego weighs 20 pounds more than Lawrence. Does this mean that Diego is overweight? Are there any factors he may not be considering? Explain.

   _____

   _____

   _____

   _____

Lesson 4.1

The Doctor Is In

Imagine that you are a doctor who treats the patients described below. Using the information provided, calculate the BMI for each patient and assess whether their BMIs are within a healthy range.

Patient A

Patient A is a 21-year-old adult male. He is 5 feet 9 inches tall and weighs 220 pounds.

1. What is Patient A's height in inches? _____

2. Use the following formula to calculate Patient A's body mass index.

BMI _____	=	Weight (lbs.) _____ Height (in.)² _____	x 730

3. Is Patient A's body mass index within a healthy range? Explain.

_____

_____

Patient B

Patient B is a 25-year-old adult female. She is 5 feet 2 inches tall and weighs 115 pounds.

4. What is Patient B's height in inches? _____

5. Use the following formula to calculate Patient B's body mass index.

BMI _____	=	Weight (lbs.) _____ Height (in.)² _____	x 730

6. Is Patient B's body mass index within a healthy range? Explain.

_____

_____

Lesson 4.2

Portion Distortion

Portion sizes have gotten larger over the past 20 years, and studies have shown that people eat more as their portion sizes increase. The below chart, based off of information from the National Heart, Lung, and Blood Institute, shows the portion sizes and calorie contents of four foods. These amounts are given for typical portions of the foods today and 20 years ago. Use the chart to answer the questions that follow.

Food	20 Years Ago		Today	
	Serving Size	Calories	Serving Size	Calories
Bagel	3"	140	6"	350
Pepperoni Pizza (large)	2 slices	500	2 slices	850
Popcorn	1 box	270	1 tub	630
Soda (regular)	6.5 oz.	85	20 oz.	250

1. Go to the MyPlate Supertracker and create a profile. Input the information requested about your age, gender, height, weight, and activity level, and then view your daily calorie allowance as calculated by this online tool. How many calories should you consume in a day? _____

2. A. If you lived 20 years ago, how many calories would you consume if you ate one serving of all of the foods in the above chart? _____

   B. What percentage of your daily calorie allowance is the number of calories consumed in question 2A? _____

3. A. How many calories would you consume if you ate one serving of all of the foods in the above chart today?_____

   B. What percentage of your daily calorie allowance is the number of calories consumed in question 3A? _____

4. If you ate the bagel for breakfast, the pizza and soda for lunch, and the popcorn for a snack today, how many calories would remain in your daily calorie allowance for dinner?
   _____

Lesson 4.2

Identify Unhealthy Eating Factors

For each of the following scenarios, identify the factors that impact each person's weight.

1. The members of Eugene's close-knit family all live within 20 minutes of each other. Several times a week, they meet for big potluck meals. Using large serving spoons, they scoop food onto their plates from the large variety of serving plates and bowls piled high with delicious foods. Many of Eugene's family members, including his parents, are overweight and obese. Recently, Eugene's doctor has told him he is overweight.

   A. What factors may be contributing to Eugene being overweight?

   _____

   _____

   B. What can Eugene do to take control of his eating patterns and weight?

   _____

   _____

2. When she is angry, sad, or anxious, Serena reaches for her favorite snack foods. After eating ice cream, chocolate pudding, or potato chips, she feels better for a short period of time. However, her bad mood returns whenever she realizes that binging on high-fat foods will only make her weight problems worse.

   A. What factors may be contributing to Serena's weight problems?

   _____

   _____

   B. What can Serena do to take control of her eating patterns and weight?

   _____

   _____

3. Chris has a busy schedule and often eats on the run. Since he stays up late most nights, he wakes up tired and late and often doesn't have time to sit down for breakfast. Instead, he will grab a candy bar and a can of soda. His after-school activities keep him away from home during dinnertime, so he eats dinner at a fast-food restaurant. Chris' coach notices the growing rolls of fat around Chris' waist, and he tells him to do something about it.

   A. What factors may be contributing to Chris' weight problem?

   _____

   _____

   B. What can Chris do to take control of his eating patterns and weight?

   _____

   _____

Lesson 4.3

Fad Diets

Find an advertisement for a weight-loss plan online, on television, or in a newspaper or magazine. Print or copy the advertisement or attach it to this page. Answer the following questions about the weight-loss plan. Prepare a presentation for your class.

1. Describe the product or service being sold.

   _____

   _____

2. According to the advertisement, how is weight loss achieved through this plan?

   _____

   _____

3. What is the target audience or market for this product or service? Explain your answer.

   _____

   _____

4. Name the company that paid for the advertisement and investigate the company's website. How does the company describe itself? Are there professional dietitians or physicians involved in the development of this product or service?

   _____

   _____

5. How much does this weight-loss plan and its products cost?

   _____

   _____

6. What evidence is given that the product or service works?

   _____

   _____

7. Does the advertisement sound "too good to be true"? Why or why not?

   _____

   _____

8. Suppose you are a healthcare provider or a dietitian. Based on what you learned in this chapter, would you recommend this product or service to a patient or client? Explain.

   _____

   _____

Lesson 4.3

Weight-Loss Goal Setting

Jeremy spends much of his free time watching television or texting his friends. He used to play hockey and soccer, but since his best friend moved away, he quit these activities. Most days he stops by a fast-food restaurant where he orders a milk shake for an after-school snack. He stays up late doing homework and watching television, so he doesn't get enough sleep. For the past four years, 15-year-old Jeremy's weight has been slowly climbing. At his last physical examination, his doctor warned that he is 15 pounds overweight and he recommended that Jeremy lose the weight before he develops any health problems. For this activity, you will help Jeremy devise a plan to lose the extra weight safely. In preparation, review the feature "How to Set a Goal" on page 23 in your textbook.

1. First, help Jeremy assess the situation by answering the following questions.

   A. Why is Jeremy's weight gain a problem?

   _____

   B. How did this problem develop?

   _____

   C. Why does Jeremy need to do something about it now?

   _____

   D. What is the healthiest approach to losing weight?

   _____

2. Write a specific and realistic goal that will help Jeremy lose 15 pounds within a reasonable timeline of 15 weeks. (*Reminder:* A person can safely lose only 1–2 pounds per week.)

   _____

   _____

3. Define the steps or actions Jeremy can take to achieve this goal.

   A. How can Jeremy break down his goal into smaller, more manageable steps that fit his 15-week time frame?

   _____

   _____

   B. List actions Jeremy can take, such as avoiding high-calorie foods and increasing his physical activity, to burn more calories.

   _____

4. While it's great that Jeremy has a plan, he now must act on his goal. Describe some support systems and resources Jeremy can put in place to make his acting on his goal more likely.

   _____

   _____

   _____

5. Jeremy should set up a system to monitor his own progress. Create a spreadsheet or checklist for Jeremy to keep track of how well he is fulfilling his goal.

6. Rewarding himself will help Jeremy stay motivated in achieving his goal. Based on what you know about Jeremy and his hobbies and interests, what rewards could he put in place for himself? At what increments should he set these rewards, to best motivate himself in his goal?

   _____

Chapter 4

Reading Practice

Reread the following passage from the textbook. Then answer the questions that follow.

How Genes Impact Weight

There are many ways in which the traits you inherit from your biological parents may influence your weight. Researchers have found 32 different genes that may influence weight, including recent evidence that suggests genes may influence obesity. Genetic factors predict a person's height and appear to predict about 40–70% of a person's BMI. Combined, these genes can have a great impact on a person's body composition. Genes also appear to influence peoples' food preferences, their metabolism, and the levels of various hormones in the body.

Genes and Food Preferences

Different people tend to have different preferences for particular types of food, and research shows that genes may influence those preferences. Some people prefer to eat foods that are high in fats such as chocolate, doughnuts, and ice cream. Other people prefer to eat salty foods such as pretzels, French fries, and potato chips.

Genes and Hormone Levels

The levels of various hormones in your body may also be influenced by your genetic makeup. Certain hormones may influence how hungry or full you feel. For example, the hormone *leptin* is an appetite-suppressant, meaning high levels of this hormone in your body leave you feeling full. Another hormone, *ghrelin*, makes you feel hungry.

Genes and Metabolism

Genes may also influence your metabolism, or the rate at which your body uses energy to carry out basic physiological processes such as breathing, digesting, and growing. Some people have a high metabolism, and their bodies use more energy to carry out these processes. As a result, they burn more calories each day. Other people have a lower metabolism, so their bodies do not burn as many calories to perform their daily activities.

_____ 1. Which of the following is influenced by genes?

A. your metabolic rate

B. your feelings of hunger

C. whether you prefer chocolate or potato chips

D. all of the above

_____ 2. The hormones leptin and ghrelin influence _____.

A. your genetic makeup

B. how hungry or full you feel

C. the rate at which your body uses energy

D. your food preferences

_____ 3. Which of the following statements about metabolism is true?

A. People have different rates of metabolism.

B. All people have the same rate of metabolism.

C. Someone with a high rate of metabolism needs less energy than someone with a low rate of metabolism.

D. none of the above

_____ 4. What is the main idea of this passage?

A. Your body needs energy to breathe, digest, and grow.

B. Some people burn more calories each day than others.

C. Researchers have found 32 different genes that may influence weight.

D. Your genes influence your weight and body composition in many ways.

Chapter 4

Practice Test

Completion: *Write the term that completes the statement in the space provided.*

1. A _____ is a record of what a person eats in a day.

2. In adults, waist circumference and waist-to-hip ratio are used to assess the distribution of _____.

3. _____ refers to a group's beliefs, values, customs, and arts.

4. Adults who are overweight were often overweight as _____.

5. Having a _____ in your bedroom raises your risks for being overweight or obese.

True/False: *Indicate whether each statement below is true or false by circling either T or F.*

T   F   6. Female bodies have a greater proportion of body fat than male bodies.

T   F   7. Genetic factors predict about 10–20% of a person's BMI.

T   F   8. Muscle and bone weigh less than fat.

T   F   9. About 80% of adults who have diabetes are also obese.

T   F   10. Someone who is overweight can suffer from malnutrition.

Multiple Choice: *Write the letter that corresponds to the correct answer in the blank space.*

_____ 11. The percentage of American adults who are _____ doubled from 1980 to 2008.
  A. overweight   C. a healthy weight
  B. underweight   D. obese

_____ 12. Breathing, digesting, and growing are examples of basic_____.
  A. biological traits   C. physiological desires
  B. physiological processes   D. cultural factors

_____ 13. The most common cause for being underweight is _____.
  A. alcohol use   C. eating disorders
  B. drug use   D. lack of access to food

_____ 14. The physical consequences of being overweight can best be predicted by an adult's _____.
  A. weight   C. distribution of weight on the body
  B. BMI   D. total body fat

_____ 15. A person's preference for particular flavors begins to form when he or she is _____.
  A. an adult   C. in the mother's womb
  B. a child   D. a toddler

(Continued)

Name _____   Date _____

Matching: *Match each key term to its definition by writing the letter of the term in the space provided.*

_____ 16. hormone that suppresses appetite

_____ 17. often unhealthy and popular for a certain time period

_____ 18. supplement that causes fluid loss from the body

_____ 19. hormone that increases appetite and leads to hunger

_____ 20. method of measuring body composition using a device to measure the thickness of a fold of fat

_____ 21. body's requirement for something

_____ 22. practice of ingesting only water for a set period of time

_____ 23. an indicator of excess body fat that is derived from a person's height and weight

_____ 24. the yearning for something that is not needed

_____ 25. ratio of fat, bone, and muscle that make up a person's body

A. body composition

B. body mass index

C. diuretic

D. fad diets

E. fasting

F. ghrelin

G. leptin

H. physiological need

I. portion size

J. psychological desire

K. skinfold test

Analyzing Data: *Using copies of the Body Mass Index Chart for Boys (Appendix A) and the Body Mass Index Chart for Girls (Appendix B) in your textbook, answer the questions below.*

26. Suppose a 15-year-old boy has a BMI of 22. Would he be underweight, at a healthy weight, overweight, or obese? _____

27. Suppose a 19-year-old girl has a BMI of 17. Would she be underweight, at a healthy weight, overweight, or obese? _____

28. Suppose a 12-year-old boy has a BMI of 22. Would he be underweight, at a healthy weight, overweight, or obese? _____

29. Suppose a 14-year-old girl has a BMI of 17. Would she be underweight, at a healthy weight, overweight, or obese? _____

30. Calculate your own BMI using the formula below.

BMI			
_____	=	Weight (lbs.) _____ ――――――――――― Height (in.)² _____	x 730

Plot your BMI on the appropriate chart and note whether you are underweight, at a healthy weight, overweight, or obese. (Remember that for some people, BMI is not an accurate indication of body composition.)

Short Answer: *On a separate sheet of paper, answer the following questions using what you have learned in this chapter.*

31. Give an example of the "all-or-nothing" mindset about eating, and explain how it can undermine weight-loss efforts.

32. Why would having good emotional and social health contribute to someone's success in his or her weight-loss efforts?

Name _____ Date _____

Media Messages about Body Types

Many factors affect body image and a person's likelihood to develop an eating disorder. As described in the textbook, many types of media, including advertisements, magazines, television programs, and images on the Internet, idealize thinness in women and muscular bodies in men. In this activity, you will find and analyze messages from several media sources about the ideal body type.

Advertisement

Find an advertisement that portrays a thin female body or a muscular male body and that implies this body type is desirable. Staple the advertisement to this page. Then answer the following questions.

1. Where did the advertisement come from?

   _____

2. What product or service is the advertisement selling?

   _____

3. What type of person is the target audience of the advertisement? Explain your answer.

   _____

4. Describe how the advertisement portrays a thin female body or a muscular male body as desirable.

   _____

   _____

   _____

   _____

Television

Identify a television show that portrays a thin female body or a muscular male body and that implies this body type is desirable. Then answer the following questions about the show.

1. What is the name of the television show and what channel is it on?

   _____

2. Who is the intended audience for the program? Explain your answer.

   _____

3. Describe how the show portrays a thin female body or a muscular male body as desirable.

   _____

   _____

   _____

Lesson 5.1

Steroids and Athletes

Some high-profile professional athletes—both male and female—use anabolic steroids to strengthen and increase the sizes of their muscles and to give themselves a competitive edge. Find a news article about an athlete who was caught using steroids and staple it to this worksheet. Then answer the questions below.

1. Who is the athlete who was caught using steroids? What sport and sports organization is he or she associated with?

   _____

   _____

   _____

   _____

2. How was the athlete "caught"?

   _____

   _____

   _____

   _____

3. Was the athlete punished or penalized for his or her use of steroids? If so, how?

   _____

   _____

   _____

   _____

4. How did being a known steroid user impact the person's reputation and career?

   _____

   _____

   _____

   _____

5. What are possible health consequences of using steroids?

   _____

   _____

   _____

   _____

Lesson 5.2

Key Terms Review

Multiple Choice: *Write the letter that corresponds to the correct answer in the blank space.*

_____ 1. The growth of fine hair all over the body as a result of starvation is called _____.

    A. constipation   C. lanugo

    B. infertility   D. osteoporosis

_____ 2. People with eating disorders experience high rates of *mortality*, or _____.

    A. illness   C. depression

    B. death   D. malnutrition

_____ 3. Experts believe that _____ factors play the largest role in the development of eating disorders.

    A. behavioral risk   C. biological and genetic

    B. physical   D. media

_____ 4. A psychological illness characterized by a serious disturbance in a person's eating behavior is called _____.

    A. an addiction   C. anxiety

    B. depression   D. an eating disorder

_____ 5. People who have anorexia nervosa can become physically unable to reproduce, a condition called _____.

    A. infertility   C. hypoglycemia

    B. lanugo   D. acid reflux disorder

_____ 6. Some people with anorexia nervosa abuse _____, which are medications that are used to aid bowel movements.

    A. creatine   C. supplements

    B. laxatives   D. anabolic steroids

_____ 7. Hypoglycemia is a deficiency of _____ in the blood.

    A. nutrients   C. insulin

    B. water   D. sugar

Matching: *Match each statement about a disease or health condition with its name. Write the letter corresponding to the disease or condition in the blank space.*

_____ 8. recurrent episodes of binge eating followed by purging

_____ 9. condition caused by a deficiency of sugar in the blood

_____ 10. acid-containing chyme moves from the lower stomach into the esophagus

_____ 11. repeatedly consuming a huge amount of food in a short period of time

_____ 12. characterized by an intense fear of gaining weight, minimal eating, and extreme weight loss

    A. acid reflux disorder

    B. anorexia nervosa

    C. binge-eating disorder

    D. bulimia nervosa

    E. constipation

    F. hypoglycemia

Lesson 5.2

Identifying Eating Disorders

The following scenarios each describe a person who has a disturbance in his or her eating behavior. Three types of eating disorders were briefly described in the textbook: anorexia nervosa, bulimia nervosa, and binge-eating disorder. For each scenario, evaluate the person's symptoms, determine which type of eating disorder he or she likely has, and explain your answer.

1. Fifteen-year-old Denise has been receiving coaching in gymnastics since she was a young girl. Her dream is to make the national team. Denise believes that she must stay small and thin to beat out her competitors. Although she is a normal weight for her size, she restricts her diet, eating only small amounts of food each day. She has become extremely thin, and she believes she needs to stay on her severely restricted diet. She has recently stopped menstruating. Which type of eating disorder does Denise most likely have? Explain your answer.

   _____

   _____

   _____

   _____

2. Michael's friends call him the "human vacuum cleaner" because of the massive amounts of food he consumes in one sitting. His room is littered with empty potato chip bags and ice cream cartons. Michael doesn't like the teasing, but he cannot stop himself from eating huge amounts of food. Michael feels powerless to stop this behavior although he may feel full. He is afraid of becoming overweight and he feels disgusted with himself. Which type of eating disorder does Michael most likely have? Explain your answer.

   _____

   _____

   _____

   _____

3. Juliana looks like any other healthy, active 16-year-old. However, she has a problem that even her best friends don't know about. When she feels anxious, she eats and eats. To get rid of the excess calories she consumes, she vomits and exercises furiously. After her eating binges, she feels guilty and angry at herself. Which type of eating disorder does Juliana most likely have? Explain your answer.

   _____

   _____

   _____

   _____

Name _____ Date _____

Improving Your Body Image

Many people, teenagers included, spend too much time focusing on the things they don't like about their bodies. This negatively affects their body images. In this exercise, you will focus on positive things about your body and yourself. If you have problems completing the lists, ask a good friend or family member for input.

1. List 10 things you like about your body—what you and other people consider to be your best features. (For example: your smile, your soft hair, or your toned arms)

_____

_____

_____

_____

_____

_____

_____

_____

_____

_____

2. List 10 everyday physical activities that your body enables you to do. (For example: walk, climb stairs, carry things, or speak)

_____

_____

_____

_____

_____

_____

_____

_____

_____

_____

3. List 10 metabolic activities that your body carries out that keep you alive. (For example: breathe, digest food, or regulate body temperature)

_____

_____

_____

_____

(Continued)

_____

_____

_____

_____

_____

4. List 5 skills or activities that your body has been trained to do, aside from everyday activities. (For example: dance, play a particular sport or instrument)

_____

_____

_____

_____

_____

5. List 10 things you like about yourself that do not involve your physical appearance. (For example: your intelligence, your ability to start a conversation, or your empathy for others)

_____

_____

_____

_____

_____

_____

_____

_____

_____

_____

6. Write a profile of yourself using the lists you created for questions 1–5.

_____

_____

_____

_____

_____

_____

_____

_____

_____

Chapter 5

Reading Practice

Reread the following passage from the textbook. Then answer the questions that follow.

Individual Therapy

Many people find that talking with a therapist is very helpful in managing a mental or emotional illness, including eating disorders. A **therapist** is a professional trained to diagnose and treat people with mental illnesses and disorders. Therapists include psychologists, psychiatrists, social workers, and counselors. Individual therapy consists of meeting one-on-one with a therapist. Therapists help their patients better understand problems that may contribute to their eating disorders. For example, people with anorexia nervosa are often perfectionists. Therapists can help these people learn to manage their drive for perfectionism in healthier ways. In addition, therapists can help people with bulimia improve their negative self-image.

Another type of individual therapy often used to treat eating disorders is **cognitive-behavioral therapy**. This type of therapy focuses on clarifying patients' distorted thoughts and behaviors regarding food, weight, and body shape. Cognitive-behavioral therapy often employs techniques to

- help patients create more normal eating patterns by encouraging them to eat slowly and to eat regular meals;

- expand the types of foods patients are comfortable eating;

- change patients' faulty beliefs about food, such as "If I gain one pound, I'll gain a hundred," and "Any sweet is instantly converted into fat;"

- help patients develop more realistic body ideals, partially by teaching them that media images are often illusions created by digitally altering and airbrushing to correct imperfections; and

- change patients' thoughts and attitudes about eating, food, and their bodies by teaching them to avoid linking their self-esteem with their weight.

_____ 1. Which type of professional is *not* a therapist?

    A. psychologist   C. psychiatrist

    B. social worker   D. primary care physician

_____ 2. In which type of therapy does the patient meet one-on-one with the therapist?

    A. individual therapy   C. family-based therapy

    B. group therapy   D. none of the above

_____ 3. Which type of therapy targets patients' faulty beliefs and thoughts, such as "I ate two cookies so I'll never be able to lose weight"?

    A. individual therapy   C. family-based therapy

    B. cognitive-behavioral therapy   D. none of the above

_____ 4. Which statement best expresses the main idea of this passage?

    A. Talking with a therapist is helpful in treating an eating disorder.   C. In individual therapy, there are many ways a therapist can help someone with an eating disorder.

    B. People with eating disorders have a negative self-image.   D. none of the above

Chapter 5

Practice Test

Completion: *Write the term that completes the statement in the space provided.*

1. Using specialized software to conceal a model's imperfections is _____.

2. A general term for psychologists, psychiatrists, social workers, and counselors is _____.

3. Some teenagers choose to have _____ to change the shapes of their noses or eyes.

4. A person with _____ eats only very small amounts of food.

5. The most common eating disorder is _____.

True/False: *Indicate whether each statement below is true or false by circling either T or F.*

T   F   6. Your body image is determined by what your body actually looks like.

T   F   7. The preference for thin girls and women in media is relatively new.

T   F   8. Treating eating disorders is difficult because patients have a relatively high rate of relapse.

T   F   9. Patterns of interaction in families are thought to influence the development of eating disorders.

T   F   10. Most teenagers do not feel self-conscious about their bodies.

Multiple Choice: *Write the letter that corresponds to the correct answer in the blank space.*

_____ 11. Why are women in leadership positions often criticized or complimented on their physical attributes?
   A. Women in leadership positions want feedback on their appearances.
   B. Women make more effort to look nice than men.
   C. Women are defined by their physical appearances more often than men are.
   D. Women appreciate and value their bodies.

_____ 12. Factors that can influence a person's body image include _____.
   A. family and peers
   B. images in the media
   C. participation in sports
   D. all of the above

_____ 13. The average woman in the United States wears a size _____.
   A. 0 to 4
   B. 6 to 10
   C. 12 to 14
   D. none of the above

_____ 14. Media images of men have become increasingly _____.
   A. muscular
   B. thin
   C. tall
   D. feminine

_____ 15. Which sport is associated with poor body image in girls?
   A. basketball
   B. soccer
   C. softball
   D. gymnastics

Name _____

Matching: *Match each key term to its definition by writing the letter of the term in the space provided.*

_____ 16. extreme concern with becoming more muscular

_____ 17. standard of beauty that does not exist in real life

_____ 18. artificial hormones that people illegally use to build muscle

_____ 19. infrequent or delayed hard, dry bowel movements

_____ 20. form of therapy that focuses on clarifying patients' distorted thoughts and behaviors

_____ 21. can be ingested to give a person's body more of a specific nutrient

_____ 22. condition in which a person is physically unable to reproduce

_____ 23. amino acid taken as a dietary supplement to build muscle mass

_____ 24. medication used to encourage and aid bowel movements

A. anabolic steroids

B. cognitive-behavioral therapy

C. constipation

D. creatine

E. dietary supplement

F. eating disorder

G. idealized image

H. infertility

I. laxative

J. muscle dysmorphia

Analyzing Data: *The table below shows the percentage of 15-year-olds who were engaged in dieting and weight-control behaviors in various countries over the course of a year. Use the data given to answer the questions that follow.*

Country	% Boys	% Girls
Hungary	11.2	36.2
USA	20.8	30.0
Canada	9.7	29.2
Italy	6.9	27.3
Germany	5.6	19.3
Spain	5.4	18.8
HBSC average	6.9	22.6

Source: Health Behavior in School-aged Children (HBSC) Study: International Report from the World Health Organization

25. What general statement can you make about the difference between these behaviors in boys and girls across all countries in the table?

_____

26. Which countries have a percentage of 15-year-old girls engaged in dieting and weight-control behaviors that is lower than the HBSC average?

_____

_____

Short Answer: *On a separate sheet of paper, answer the following questions using what you have learned in this chapter.*

27. Does a person's happiness hinge on how he or she looks? Explain your answer.

28. Should extremely thin models be banned from fashion shows, advertisements, and publications in the United States? Explain your answer.

(Continued)

Lesson 6.1

Health and History

A family history is a record of a disease's occurrence within a family. If someone in a person's family has had a disease, then that person is more likely to develop the same disease. Even though you are "stuck" with the genes and family history that you have, physical activity can help reduce your risk for some family diseases. In this activity, you will discover what diseases you are at risk for developing and will then determine how physical activity can help reduce your risk. To find out which diseases you are at risk of developing, assemble a family history. Interview your family members about diseases common in your family. Then, using your knowledge about these diseases and about the benefits of physical activity, explain what kinds of physical activity you could engage in to reduce your risk of developing each disease.

1. Disease: _____

   Family history: _____

   Physical activity and benefits: _____

   _____

2. Disease: _____

   Family history: _____

   Physical activity and benefits: _____

   _____

3. Disease: _____

   Family history: _____

   Physical activity and benefits: _____

   _____

4. Disease: _____

   Family history: _____

   Physical activity and benefits: _____

   _____

5. Disease: _____

   Family history: _____

   Physical activity and benefits: _____

   _____

Name _____ Date _____

Charting Your Physical Activity

Statistics show that only 35% of American adults engage in physical activity five times a week. Are you part of that 35%? To find out, you will record your physical activity for five days in the chart below.

During the next five days, list times when you engage in sedentary activity and times when you engage in physical activity—be honest! After the five days, count how many times you were physically active and how many times you were sedentary. Did you engage in physical activity all five days?

If you did not engage in at least one physical activity each day, examine your chart to determine when you could fit physical activity into your schedule next week. Using a red pen, "revise" your schedule for the week so that it includes more physical activity. Then try charting your activity for the next five days after that. Finally, answer the questions at the bottom of this page.

My Five-Day Chart				
Day One	**Day Two**	**Day Three**	**Day Four**	**Day Five**

1. Which sedentary activities do you think you could delete from your schedule?

   _____

   _____

2. Which physical activities would you be most interested in including in your schedule?

   _____

   _____

3. During the second week when you scheduled a physical activity each day, did you notice any difference in your mood, energy, or concentration? Explain.

   _____

   _____

Lesson 6.2

Healthy Weight Control

Judy and her groups of friends want to lose weight and they know that one of the many health benefits of physical activity is improved weight control. They also know they must engage in a certain amount of physical activity before they will see any weight-loss results. To work off one pound of body weight, a person must burn about 3,500 calories, but Judy and her friends have busy schedules with extracurricular activities in the afternoons.

The chart below shows how many calories a person would burn during 30 minutes of physical activity based on intensity and body weight. Using this chart, answer the questions that follow for Judy and each of her friends.

Approximate Calories Burned for Different Physical Activities

Moderate Physical Activity	Calories Burned in 30 Minutes of Activity				
	100-lb. person	120-lb. person	135-lb. person	150-lb. person	200-lb. person
hiking climbing stairs	136	164	184	205	273
gardening softball	114	136	153	170	227
calisthenics mopping scrubbing floors	102	123	138	153	205
bicycling (< 10 mph) brisk walking (> 3 mph)	91	109	123	136	182
weight lifting (light workout)	68	82	92	102	136
Vigorous Physical Activity	**Calories Burned in 30 Minutes of Activity**				
	100-lb. person	120-lb. person	135-lb. person	150-lb. person	200-lb. person
rock climbing (ascending)	250	300	338	375	500
running (10 min. mile) bicycling (>10 mph)	227	273	300	341	455
football tennis (singles) calisthenics (push-ups, sit-ups) jumping rope	182	218	245	273	364
soccer rollerblading	159	191	215	239	318
swimming basketball (half-court) shoveling snow	136	164	184	205	273
dancing (vigorous)	125	150	169	187	250

Name _____

1. **Judy:** weight: 200 lbs.; healthy weight goal: 160 lbs. (-40 lbs.); schedule conflicts: band practice every afternoon and music lessons Saturday morning

   A. How can Judy fit physical activity into her busy schedule?

   _____

   B. What *moderate* physical activity can Judy engage in?

   _____

   C. How many hours of physical activity are required to work off one pound?

   _____

   D. How many hours of physical activity are required to reach Judy's weight-loss goal?

   _____

2. **Adam:** *weight: 120 lbs.; healthy weight goal: 100 lbs. (-20 lbs.); schedule conflicts: student council duties every Thursday afternoon and some weekends*

   A. How can Adam fit physical activity into his busy schedule?

   _____

   B. What *vigorous* physical activity can Adam engage in?

   _____

   C. How many hours of physical activity are required to work off one pound?

   _____

   D. How many hours of physical activity are required to reach Adam's weight-loss goal?

   _____

3. **Jalisa:** *weight: 135 lbs.; healthy weight goal: 115 lbs. (-20 lbs.); schedule conflicts: volunteers at the local library all day on Saturdays*

   A. How can Jalisa fit physical activity into her busy schedule?

   _____

   B. What *vigorous* physical activity can Jalisa engage in?

   _____

   C. How many hours of physical activity are required to work off one pound?

   _____

   D. How many hours of physical activity are required to reach Jalisa's weight-loss goal?

   _____

4. **Malcolm:** *weight: 200 lbs.; healthy weight goal: 150 lbs. (-50 lbs.); schedule conflicts: Tuesday afternoon book club meetings, various club duties on the weekends*

   A. How can Malcolm fit physical activity into his busy schedule?

   _____

   B. What *moderate* physical activity can Malcolm engage in?

   _____

   C. How many hours of physical activity are required to work off one pound?

   _____

   D. How many hours of physical activity are required to reach Malcolm's weight-loss goal?

   _____

Lesson 6.2

Key Terms Review

Multiple Choice: *Write the letter that corresponds to the correct answer in the blank space.*

_____ 1. Activity involving the use of oxygen to fuel body processes is known as _____.
   A. anaerobic
   B. health-related
   C. aerobic
   D. skill-related

_____ 2. _____ fitness is the type of fitness used to easily perform daily activities.
   A. Range of motion
   B. Skill-related
   C. Overload
   D. Health-related

_____ 3. Your _____ is determined by the elasticity of your muscles and connective tissues.
   A. flexibility
   B. agility
   C. intensity
   D. speed

_____ 4. The _____ include strength and flexibility.
   A. range of motion procedures
   B. speed exercises
   C. components of fitness
   D. training principles

_____ 5. The ability to quickly change the body's momentum and direction is called _____.
   A. agility
   B. speed
   C. flexibility
   D. intensity

_____ 6. The term _____ describes how efficiently the cardiovascular and respiratory systems deliver oxygen to the muscles during prolonged physical activity.
   A. *agility*
   B. *cardiorespiratory fitness*
   C. *intensity*
   D. *skill-related fitness*

_____ 7. _____ describes how far a joint can move in a particular direction.
   A. Flexibility
   B. Aerobic exercise
   C. Range of motion
   D. Agility

_____ 8. _____ in a number of different activities can improve performance in a sport and reduce the risk of injury.
   A. Skill training
   B. Health training
   C. Motion training
   D. Cross training

_____ 9. In _____ exercise, activity occurs in the absence of oxygen.
   A. skill-related
   B. anaerobic
   C. health-related
   D. aerobic

_____ 10. _____ fitness improves a person's performance in a particular sport.
   A. Health-related
   B. Cardiorespiratory
   C. Skill-related
   D. Training

_____ 11. The quality measured by how much energy the body uses per minute during physical activity is known as _____.
   A. intensity
   B. speed
   C. flexibility
   D. agility

_____ 12. While performing aerobic exercises that lead to optimal cardiorespiratory fitness, you should aim for your _____.
   A. optimal range of motion
   B. target heart rate
   C. highest level of flexibility
   D. skill exercise goal

Matching: *Match each statement about a training principle with the correct training principle. Write the letter corresponding to the training principle in the blank space.*

A. FITT factors should be increased over time to improve fitness.

B. A gradual increase of a physical demand on the body will improve fitness.

C. Exercising a particular component leads to improvements in the fitness of only that component.

_____ 13. overload principle

_____ 14. specificity principle

_____ 15. progression principle

Name _____ Date _____

Adding It All Up

The chart below lists different types of physical activity based on what they achieve (such as strengthening bones or providing a vigorous workout). Consider what you want to achieve in your own personal fitness plan and choose at least three of these activities to include in a weeklong plan for yourself. Use your five-day chart from the "Lesson 6.1: Charting Your Physical Activity" exercise to review what physical activities you have or are currently engaging in, and to determine space in your schedule. If you want to achieve a healthy weight goal, review the chart in the "Lesson 6.2: Healthy Weight Control" exercise to determine how many calories you need to burn in a week. Once you have chosen three or more activities, write them in your new five-day chart. Also record any active or sedentary behaviors you are still engaging in from the five-day chart in "Lesson 6.1: Charting Your Physical Activity."

Physical Activities You Can Do to Increase Fitness

Moderate-Intensity Activities	Vigorous-Intensity Activities	Muscle-Strengthening Activities	Bone-Strengthening Activities
walking briskly; raking leaves; biking (slower than 10 miles per hour); skateboarding; mowing the lawn; basketball; volleyball; hiking; rollerblading; canoeing; shoveling snow; doubles tennis	soccer; jumping rope; martial arts, such as karate, singles tennis; field or ice hockey; aerobics; cheerleading; gymnastics; jogging or running; swimming laps; rollerblading or skating at a brisk pace; cross-country skiing; football; basketball; soccer; aerobic dancing; biking (10 miles per hour or faster); hiking uphill or with a heavy backpack	push-ups; sit-ups; rock climbing; using weight machines; lifting handheld weights; using resistance bands	jumping rope; running; gymnastics; volleyball; tennis; basketball

My Five-Day Chart

Day One	Day Two	Day Three	Day Four	Day Five

Name _____ Date _____

Fitness That Fits You

Fitness plans are personal. Each person will want to achieve something different, and each person should exercise how he or she is most comfortable. What works for you might not work for someone else. What works for your best friend might not fit what you need.

Using online or print resources, research the different fitness methods listed below. For each method of fitness, answer the following questions and record them in the chart below.

What is involved in this type of fitness? How much would this fitness method cost? How much time would this method take out of my week? Is the method solitary, or does it involve joining a team or group?

Once you have answered these questions and have researched each method thoroughly, decide whether each method would "fit" you and explain why or why not. Choosing fitness methods that work for you will help you in sticking to a personal fitness plan.

Fitness Method	Does It Fit *Me*?	Explain
Weight lifting What's involved: Cost: Time: Solitary or group-oriented?		
Jogging What's involved: Cost: Time: Solitary or group-oriented?		
Yoga What's involved: Cost: Time: Solitary or group-oriented?		
Cardio exercise with video guidance What's involved: Cost: Time: Solitary or group-oriented?		
Other: What's involved: Cost: Time: Solitary or group-oriented?		

Name _____ Date _____

Be a Smart Fitness Consumer

For some physical activities, fitness equipment or products are required. Football players need helmets, runners need shoes that protect their feet, and everyone needs to stay hydrated while exercising. Research the equipment and products that you, your school, or other people you know use. Then, based on your own experience or on discussions with others who use these products, assess whether each piece of equipment or product is as effective as its company might claim.

1. *Football helmets (the brand used at your school)*

   Name the brand of football helmet used at your school:

   _____

   Claims made about this product:

   _____

   _____

   Opinions of the players and coaches:

   _____

   Alternative brands or products:

   _____

2. *Running shoes (a brand used by you or someone you know)*

   Name the brand of running shoes that you or someone you know uses:

   _____

   Claims made about this product:

   _____

   _____

   Opinions of those who use the product:

   _____

   Alternative brands or products:

   _____

3. *Water or sports drinks (a brand used by someone you know)*

   Name the brand of water or sports drinks that you or someone you know uses:

   _____

   Claims made about this product:

   _____

   _____

   Opinions of those who use this product:

   _____

   Alternative brands or products:

   _____

Chapter 6

Reading Practice

Reread the following passage from the textbook. Then answer the questions that follow.

Improving Your Physical Fitness

We often think of the terms *physical activity* and *exercise* as meaning the same thing. A difference does exist, however, between these two terms. **Exercise**—meaning a type of physical activity that is planned, structured, and purposeful—is actually just one type of physical activity. *Exercise* could describe the cycle of exercises you do in PE class, a varsity sports team's daily practice, or running every day to prepare for a half-marathon.

The term **physical activity** is broader because it includes structured exercise as well as other activities that use energy. Biking to school, playing Frisbee with friends, and dancing to music alone in your bedroom are not what we would typically call *exercise*, but they are all definitely *physical activity*.

Deciding to exercise is a good lifestyle choice if you want to be physically fit. You do not need to engage in structured exercise, however, to improve your fitness level. Your health and fitness can benefit from many different types of physical activity.

If you don't currently get regular physical activity of any kind, you may find it difficult to get started. Many easy strategies exist for you to begin and maintain a fitness program.

_____ 1. Exercise is planned, structured, and _____.
   A. uses equipment
   B. purposeful
   C. done in a group
   D. fast-paced

_____ 2. Biking to school and _____ alone in your bedroom are both examples of physical activity.
   A. sleeping
   B. writing
   C. dancing
   D. reading

_____ 3. Which of the following would be considered *exercise*?
   A. drills with your sports team
   B. playing catch with your dog
   C. walking your dog
   D. playing "tag" with friends

_____ 4. Which of the following is an example of physical activity?
   A. lifting weights
   B. mowing the lawn
   C. playing Frisbee with friends
   D. all of the above

Chapter 6

Practice Test

Completion: *Write the term that completes the statement in the space provided.*

1. Many people spend much of their day engaging in _____ behavior rather than physical activity.

2. Physical activity can lower your risk for developing certain _____.

3. Some people use the acronym _____ to help them focus on the key factors in physical activity.

4. The _____ states that you must put a greater demand on your body to improve it.

5. It is essential to drink lots of _____ before, during, and even after engaging in physical activity.

True/False: *Indicate whether each statement below is true or false by circling either T or F.*

T   F   6. A calorie deficit leads to weight gain.

T   F   7. People who engage in regular physical activity experience a better quality of sleep than those who do not exercise.

T   F   8. Muscular strength is the ability of a muscle to exert force against resistance.

T   F   9. Skill-related fitness means fitness that is used to perform daily activities.

T   F   10. You should avoid exercising outside when it is hot or humid.

Multiple Choice: *Write the letter that corresponds to the correct answer in the blank space.*

_____ 11. The body's ability to meet daily physical demands is _____.
   A. flexibility
   B. fitness
   C. agility
   D. exercise

_____ 12. Which of the following is true of fitness programs?
   A. All fitness programs should consist of the same types of physical activity.
   B. A fitness program should be far too difficult for your current level of fitness.
   C. A fitness program should match up well with your daily life and interests.
   D. A fitness program should be private and should not be shared with your friends or family.

_____ 13. An easy way to monitor the intensity of physical activity is to check your _____.
   A. pulse
   B. sweat levels
   C. breathing
   D. endurance

_____ 14. _____ is a combination of strength and speed.
   A. Coordination
   B. Agility
   C. Balance
   D. Power

_____ 15. Although sports drinks can help you stay hydrated, _____ is an even better option.
   A. soda
   B. chocolate milk
   C. an energy drink
   D. coffee

Name _____

Analyzing Data: *The graph shown here represents health patterns—including patterns of activity, screen time, and diet—for 10,000 students between 11 and 16 years of age. These patterns are classified as typical, unhealthful, or healthful. Study the data in this graph and then answer the questions that follow.*

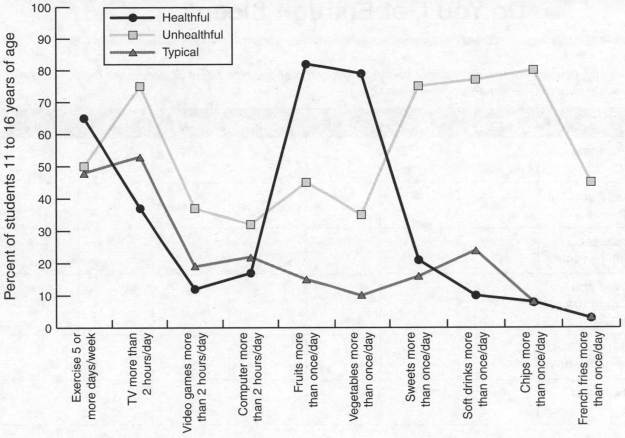

Source: National Institute of Health (NIH)

16. What percentage of typical students engage in exercise five or more days a week?

_____

17. Which factor presents the largest percentage difference between healthful students and unhealthful students? What does this tell you about the importance of that health factor?

_____

18. Which factor(s) presents the smallest percentage difference(s) between unhealthful students and healthful students? How does this challenge what you may have thought before about healthful patterns of activity?

_____

Short Answer: *On a separate sheet of paper, answer the following questions using what you have learned in this chapter.*

19. What are some simple ways that you can incorporate more physical activity into your daily life? Remember that physical activity does not have to be structured.

20. What are some of your personal fitness goals? Based on those goals, what are the best types of physical activity for you to engage in?

Name _____ Date _____

Do You Get Enough Sleep?

In this activity, you will determine whether you get the recommended nine hours of sleep each night. For one week, track your sleep schedule in the chart below.

	Mon	Tues	Wed	Thurs	Fri	Sat	Sun
When did you go to bed?							
When did you fall asleep?							
Did you sleep through the night?							
When did you wake up in the morning?							
How did you feel upon waking up?							
Total hours of sleep:							

1. On which days did you get nine or more hours of sleep? On which days did you get less than nine hours of sleep?

   _____

   _____

   _____

2. Calculate the average number of hours of sleep you got during the week. Show your work.

   _____

   _____

   _____

3. On nights when you slept less than the recommended number of hours, how did you feel when you woke up the next morning? How did you feel the next day?

   _____

   _____

   _____

4. Based on your sleep log, how many hours of sleep do you need to feel your best the next day? What time would you need to go to bed to get this amount of sleep?

   _____

   _____

   _____

Name _____

5. Based on your data and observations, do you agree with the recommendation that teenagers get at least nine hours of sleep each night? Explain.

_____

_____

_____

6. On nights when you didn't get adequate sleep, explain why this happened. For example, did you wake up in the middle of the night with a nightmare, did you have difficulty falling asleep, or were you up too late?

_____

_____

_____

If you don't get the sleep you need, list three steps you can take to remedy the problem. Consult your textbook for ideas. Then implement these steps and record your progress in the chart below. Afterward, answer the questions that follow.

	Check Box for Each Step You Complete						
	Mon	Tues	Wed	Thurs	Fri	Sat	Sun
1.							
2.							
3.							
Total hours of sleep:							
How did you feel upon waking up?							

7. Did taking the three steps help you get more sleep?

_____

_____

_____

8. When you took these three steps, did you feel more rested the next morning and the next day? Explain.

_____

_____

_____

Name _____   Date _____

Sleep Deprivation and Driving

According to the National Highway Traffic Safety Administration (NHTSA), sleep deprivation may contribute to 30–40% of all heavy truck crashes. Long-distance truck drivers who work overnight or who work long, irregular hours are more susceptible than other drivers to the effects of sleep deprivation. These effects include decreased alertness, decreased reaction time, and increased microsleeps (brief episodes of sleep that last from a fraction of a second to 10 seconds). The graph below depicts the times of day during which truck drivers are most susceptible to the effects of drowsiness. This susceptibility is associated with the body's circadian rhythm, the natural pattern of physiological processes that occurs within a 24-hour period. As fatigue increases, alertness decreases. Examine the graph. Then answer the questions that follow.

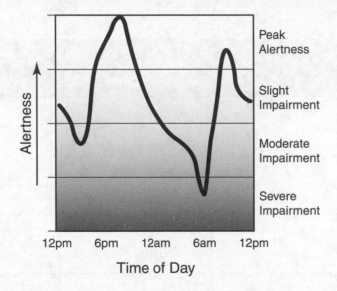

Source: Dr. Nancy Grugle and Brooks Rugemer, Robson Forensics:
"Sleep Deprivation and Fatigue in Commercial Truck Crashes" (January 31, 2014).

1. At approximately what time of day do truck drivers experience peak alertness?

   _____

2. Around what time of day do truck drivers experience their second highest peak in alertness?

   _____

3. Between what hours of the day does driver alertness dip from slight impairment to moderate impairment before rising again?

   _____

4. Between what hours of the day is moderate impairment in driver alertness most evident before diving toward severe impairment?

   _____

5. Generally, what is the worst time of day for truck drivers to be on the road?

   _____

6. Based on the data in this graph, what can you conclude about when truck-driver crashes are likely to occur due to sleep deprivation?

   _____

Lesson 7.2

The Science behind Sleep

Multiple Choice: *Write the letter that corresponds to the correct answer in the blank space.*

_____ 1. What is the term for the naturally occurring physical, behavioral, and mental changes in the body that typically follow the 24-hour cycle of the sun?

      A. suprachiasmatic cadence   C. somnolence periodicity

      B. circadian rhythm   D. hypothalamic hibernation

_____ 2. This group of nerve cells in the brain controls many physiological responses in the body, including the sleep-wake cycle, body temperature, hormone levels, and brain wave activity.

      A. supraneural regulators   C. suprachiasmatic nucleus (SCN)

      B. supraneural hub   D. hypothalamic nucleus (HTN)

_____ 3. _____ is a type of fatigue that people feel after changing time zones when they travel.

      A. Jet drag   C. Jet delay

      B. Jet lag   D. Jet resistance

_____ 4. Which of the following hormones released by the pineal gland increases feelings of relaxation and fatigue?

      A. melanostatin   C. melanin

      B. pheomelanin   D. melatonin

_____ 5. The body's biological clock follows the cycle of _____.

      A. semiregular variable stars   C. the moon

      B. periodic comets   D. the sun

_____ 6. During this stage of sleep, you drift in and out of sleep and can be easily awakened.

      A. Stage 1   C. Stage 3

      B. Stage 2   D. Stage 4

_____ 7. During this active stage of sleep, your breathing grows irregular, heart rate and blood pressure rise, your eyes dart about beneath your eyelids, and your muscles are temporarily paralyzed.

      A. Stage 2   C. Stage 4

      B. Stage 3   D. REM sleep

_____ 8. During this stage of sleep, muscle activity and eye movements completely stop, and you become difficult to awaken.

      A. Stage 2   C. Stage 4

      B. Stage 3   D. REM sleep

_____ 9. During what stage of sleep can bursts of intense brain activity called *spindles* occur?

      A. Stage 1   C. Stage 3

      B. Stage 2   D. Stage 4

_____ 10. Which stage of sleep marks the transitional stage between light sleep and deep sleep, when brain wave activity slows?

      A. Stage 1   D. Stage 4

      B. Stage 2

      C. Stage 3

(Continued)

_____ 11. From Stage 1 through REM sleep, a complete sleep cycle lasts approximately _____ minutes.
   A. 45 to 90   C. 60 to 120
   B. 60 to 90   D. 90 to 110

_____ 12. During which stage of sleep are the brain regions used for learning stimulated?
   A. Stage 3   C. REM sleep
   B. Stage 4   D. none of the above

_____ 13. Why might infants spend more time in REM sleep than adults?
   A. REM sleep is thought to be important for normal brain development during infancy.
   B. Infants have more active brains than adults.
   C. The body's need for REM sleep decreases with age.
   D. Brain activity diminishes with age.

Matching: *Match each stage of sleep to its characteristics by writing the letter of the stage in the blank space.*

_____ 14. This transitional stage occurs between light sleep and deep sleep.   A. Stage 1

_____ 15. In this stage, your body temperature starts to drop, and your heart rate slows.   B. Stage 2

                                                                                                  C. Stage 3
_____ 16. During this stage of deep sleep, muscular activity stops, and you become difficult to awaken.   D. Stage 4

                                                                                                  E. REM sleep
_____ 17. During this stage of sleep, many people experience a sensation of falling, which may jolt their bodies awake.

_____ 18. In this active stage of sleep, breathing grows irregular, heart rate and blood pressure rise, the eyes dart about beneath the eyelids, and temporary muscular paralysis occurs.

Lesson 7.3

You Be the Doctor

For this activity, imagine that you are a doctor helping patients who are struggling with common sleeping problems. Analyze each scenario and determine which sleeping problem fits the symptoms. Explain your answers.

1. Joe is a 53-year-old man who comes in with his wife, Juliette. Joe says he is frequently irritable and depressed. He has had several minor accidents at work and at home, including a fall that broke his leg. Juliette complains that Joe's loud snoring has been getting worse and that he seems to stop breathing dozens of time each night. Which common sleeping problem do you think Joe has? Explain your answer.

    _____

    _____

    _____

    _____

2. Aliah is a 15-year-old girl who comes in with her mother. Aliah's mother says she has found Aliah walking around her room in the middle of the night. Although she appears awake, Aliah responds to questions with incoherent muttering. She eventually returns to her bed. Which common sleeping problem do you think Aliah has? Explain your answer.

    _____

    _____

    _____

    _____

3. Seventeen-year-old Nathan complains that he is exhausted. Since his parents told him they were divorcing, he has been upset and has had difficulty sleeping. When he gets into bed, he tosses and turns, even when he's very tired. It can be hours before he finally falls asleep. Which common sleeping problem do you think Nathan has? Explain your answer.

    _____

    _____

    _____

    _____

4. Marcus frequently wakes up with a sore jaw and a headache. The muscles in his face and neck frequently hurt. He notices the soreness is worse during periods of stress, such as during the end of the semester when multiple projects are due. His dentist told him he has several cracked molars that need to be fixed. Which common sleeping problem do you think Marcus has? Explain your answer.

    _____

    _____

    _____

    _____

Chapter 7

Reading Practice

Reread the following passage from the textbook. Then answer the questions on the next page.

Regular changes occur in your body on a daily basis. For example, your body temperature, blood pressure, and levels of different hormones rise and fall regularly. *Circadian rhythms* are naturally occurring physical, behavioral, and mental changes in the body that typically follow the 24-hour cycle of the sun. For example, the body temperature drops during the night and rises during the day.

Figure 7.3

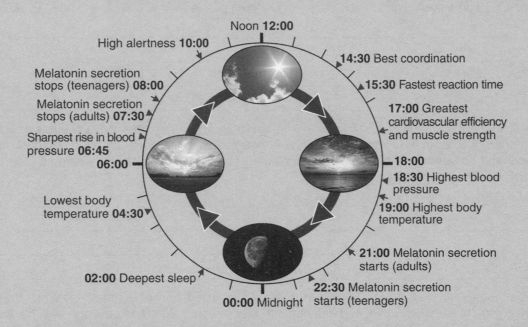

The Body's Biological Clock

Most circadian rhythms are controlled by the body's master biological "clock." This clock, called the *suprachiasmatic nucleus (SCN)*, is a group of nerve cells in a part of the brain called the *hypothalamus*. The SCN controls many physiological responses in the body, including the sleep-wake cycle, body temperature, hormone levels, and brain wave activity.

Sleep and Circadian Rhythm

Your body's biological clock determines when you feel tired and when you feel awake. There are generally two periods of the day during which the body feels like sleeping—at night and in the early part of the afternoon, between 1 p.m. and 3 p.m. In many cultures, the early part of the afternoon is a dedicated rest time, or *siesta*.

The SCN works in two ways to regulate sleep. First, it monitors the amount of light in the environment. It leads the body to be more active when there is more light and less active when there is less light. The SCN also causes the pineal gland to release the hormone *melatonin* during the late evening, which increases feelings of relaxation and sleepiness, and signals that it is time to go to sleep. Compared with adults, teenagers' melatonin is typically released later in the evening and remains at high levels in the blood until later in the morning. This biological difference contributes to the difficulty teenagers have falling asleep earlier in the evening and waking up early the next morning.

Name _____ Date _____

_____ 1. Which of the following processes is *not* controlled by your body's biological clock?
   A. brain wave activity
   B. cognitive activity
   C. sleep-wake cycle
   D. body temperature

_____ 2. Why do teenagers tend to have difficulty falling asleep earlier in the evening and waking up early the next morning?
   A. In teenagers, melatonin is typically released later in the evening and remains at high levels in the blood until later in the morning.
   B. The suprachiasmatic nucleus (SCN) in the hypothalamus of the teenage brain is not yet fully developed.
   C. The teenage brain generally has lower levels of melatonin.
   D. both A and C

Refer to Figure 7.3 to answer the questions that follow.

_____ 3. At what time is your body temperature typically the highest during a 24-hour period?
   A. 3:00 p.m.
   B. 5:00 p.m.
   C. 7:00 p.m.
   D. 9:00 p.m.

_____ 4 . When does the body generally experience the fastest reaction times?
   A. 3:30 p.m.
   B. 4:30 p.m.
   C. 5:30 p.m.
   D. 6:30 p.m.

_____ 5. At what time does melatonin secretion begin in teenagers?
   A. 9:00 p.m.
   B. 9:30 p.m.
   C. 10:00 p.m.
   D. 10:30 p.m.

_____ 6. According to the data in this figure, when would be the *optimal* time to go swimming, lift weights, or run five miles?
   A. 5:00 p.m.
   B. 6:30 p.m.
   C. 7:00 p.m.
   D. none of the above

Chapter 7

Practice Test

Completion: *Write the term that completes the statement in the space provided.*

1. _____ is a shortage of sleep that leads to tiredness and may lead to other health problems.

2. The part of the brain that regulates appetite and the consumption of energy is called the _____.

3. The _____ is a group of nerve cells in a part of the brain that controls many physiological responses in the body, including the sleep-wake cycle, body temperature, hormone levels, and brain wave activity.

4. _____ have a genetic mutation that regulates their sleep-wake cycles; they can function on less sleep than other people.

5. The _____ is the naturally occurring physical, behavioral, and mental changes in the body that typically follow the 24-hour cycle of the sun.

6. _____ is a hormone released by the pineal gland that increases feelings of relaxation and tiredness.

7. Your body's _____ determines when you feel tired and when you feel awake.

8. During sleep, the brain creates important connections between _____ that can improve memory and learning.

9. The _____ system regulates hormone levels in the body.

10. _____ is a condition in which the body is unable to fall asleep or stay asleep.

True/False: *Indicate whether each statement below is true or false by circling either T or F.*

T   F   11. Chronic insomnia is usually a symptom or side effect of another problem, such as a medical condition, sleep disorder, or substance use.

T   F   12. Bruxism is a disorder in which people experience sleeplessness due to sensations of crawling, prickling, or tingling in the lower legs and feet.

T   F   13. Parasomnia is a classification of sleep disorders that occur when people are partially, but not completely, aroused from sleep.

T   F   14. Everyone who snores has sleep apnea, a serious disorder in which one stops breathing for short periods of time during sleep.

T   F   15. The term *narcolepsy* is a synonym for *insomnia*.

T   F   16. In each successive sleep cycle, REM sleep periods get longer while deep sleep periods get shorter.

Multiple Choice: *Write the letter that corresponds to the correct answer in the blank space.*

_____ 17. Which of the following is *not* an example of parasomnia?

    A. nightmares   C. apnea

    B. sleepwalking   D. bruxism

_____ 18. Which of the following methods is used to treat sleep apnea?

    A. continuous positive airway pressure (CPAP) therapy

    B. stimulants and antidepressants

    C. sleeping pills

    D. continuous positive tracheal dilation (CPTD) therapy

_____ 19. Bruxism involves which of the following behaviors during sleep?

    A. sleepwalking

    B. grinding of the teeth

    C. "sleep-eating"

    D. talking in one's sleep

_____ 20. This disorder causes people to have frequent "sleep attacks" during the day, even if they have had a normal amount of nighttime sleep.

    A. insomnia

    B. parasomnia

    C. narcohypnia

    D. narcolepsy

_____ 21. Which of the following substances produces a temporary increase in activity in the body, making it difficult to sleep?

    A. stimulants

    B. depressants

    C. opioids

    D. analgesics

_____ 22. Scientific studies have shown that people who routinely fail to get enough sleep are more likely to develop which of the following health conditions?

    A. cardiovascular disease

    B. cardiac arrhythmias

    C. coronary heart disease

    D. all of the above

_____ 23. Which of the following substances is an amino acid that aids the body in producing chemicals that help you sleep?

    A. melatonin

    B. melanostatin

    C. tryptophan

    D. tryptase

_____ 24. Which substance listed below is *not* a stimulant?

    A. caffeinated coffee

    B. milk

    C. chocolate

    D. energy drinks

Matching: *Match each key term to its definition by writing the letter of the term in the space provided.*

_____ 25. the cells that make up nerve tissue

_____ 26. the part of the brain that regulates appetite and energy consumption

_____ 27. naturally occurring physical, behavioral, and mental changes in the body that typically follow the 24-hour cycle of the sun

_____ 28. a hormone released by the pineal gland that increases feelings of relaxation and drowsiness

_____ 29. a cluster of nerve cells in the hypothalamus that controls sleep, body temperature, hormone levels, and brain activity

_____ 30. clenching of the teeth; a common behavior during sleep

_____ 31. an amino acid that aids the body in manufacturing chemicals that cause sleep

_____ 32. a type of therapy in which a machine is used to open the airways during sleep

_____ 33. a disorder characterized by "sleep attacks" in which a person suddenly falls asleep at various times during the day

_____ 34. classification of sleep disorders that occur when people are partially, but not completely, aroused from sleep

_____ 35. inability to fall asleep or stay asleep

A. bruxism

B. circadian rhythm

C. continuous positive airway pressure (CPAP) therapy

D. hypothalamus

E. insomnia

F. melatonin

G. narcolepsy

H. neurons

I. parasomnia

J. suprachiasmatic nucleus (SCN)

K. tryptophan

Lesson 8.1

Key Concepts Review

Multiple Choice: *Write the letter that corresponds to the correct answer in the blank space.*

_____ 1. Which structure makes up the outer layer of the skin?
  A. dermis
  B. hypodermis
  C. epidermis
  D. melanin

_____ 2. Which of the following is *not* a function of the skin?
  A. protects the muscles, bones, ligaments, and internal organs
  B. serves as a barrier to bacteria, viruses, and other foreign substances
  C. regulates body temperature
  D. regulates hormonal activity

_____ 3. What kind of medical doctor specializes in treatment of the skin?
  A. dermatologist
  B. ophthalmologist
  C. endocrinologist
  D. pathologist

_____ 4. Fingernails and toenails are made up of layers of a hard protein called _____.
  A. melanin
  B. keratin
  C. cuticle
  D. none of the above

_____ 5. Which of the following determines whether your hair is straight, curly, thick, or thin?
  A. collagen
  B. elastin
  C. hair follicles
  D. lipocytes

_____ 6. Which structures or substances are *not* found in the hypodermis?
  A. blood vessels
  B. fat
  C. nerve endings
  D. melanin

_____ 7. Which structure of the skin contains hair follicles?
  A. epidermis
  B. dermis
  C. hypodermis
  D. sweat gland ducts

_____ 8. Dead skin that flakes off the scalp is known as -____.
  A. dandruff
  B. acne
  C. lice
  D. sebum

_____ 9. Which of the following may be a sign of illness or disorder?
  A. nail discoloration
  B. curled nails
  C. redness and swelling around the nail
  D. all of the above

_____ 10. Which of the following is *not* an example of how lice can be transmitted?
  A. direct head-to-head contact
  B. sharing of brushes or combs
  C. sharing of hats or headgear
  D. contact with human blood

Matching: *Match each definition to its term by writing the letter corresponding to the term in the blank space.*

_____ 11. oil produced by glands in the skin

_____ 12. outermost layer of the skin

_____ 13. middle layer of the skin, which contains hair follicles

_____ 14. substance that gives skin its pigment

_____ 15. innermost layer of the skin, which contains fat, blood vessels, and nerve endings

A. epidermis

B. dermis

C. hypodermis

D. melanin

E. sebum

Name _____ Date _____

How Is Your Hygiene?

Read each of the following personal hygiene and basic healthcare behaviors that influence your overall health. Write the number that best describes your hygiene practices. Then total your score. The higher your score, the better you are at taking care of your body's hygiene.

1—Never

2—Once in a while

3—Sometimes

4—Most of the time

5—Always

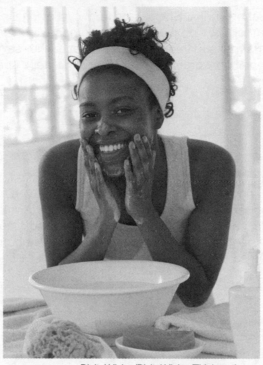

Digital Vision/Digital Vision/Thinkstock.com

_____ 1. I take a bath or shower.

_____ 2. I use a deodorant and/or antiperspirant.

_____ 3. I wear clean clothes.

_____ 4. I wash my face twice a day.

_____ 5. I wash my hair regularly to keep it clean.

_____ 6. I do not have dandruff.

_____ 7. I do not bite my fingernails.

_____ 8. I brush my teeth at least twice a day.

_____ 9. I floss my teeth every day.

_____ 10. I replace my toothbrush every three months.

_____ **Total Score**

Lesson 8.2

Prescribe the Remedy

For each scenario described below, imagine that you are a doctor. Briefly explain the cause of each patient's physical problem and state the remedy or treatment that you recommend. Indicate whether or not you think a referral to a specialist is necessary.

1. Lindsay is a 17-year-old high school junior. She suffers from cystic acne, a particularly severe form of acne. Lindsay is highly active; she participates on the school track team, and she notes that she "always seems to be sweating." She often wears makeup in an attempt to conceal her severe acne breakouts, and the makeup seems to make her condition worse. She asks you what steps she can take to prevent more acne outbreaks.

   _____

   _____

   _____

2. Liam is a 56-year-old advertising account manager. Over the past month, he has suffered from dry, itchy skin that has become swollen and red. Although he tries not to scratch his skin, he finds himself doing so because the itchiness is unbearable at times. As a result, he has developed small, infected patches on his skin. Liam has a stressful career that demands long hours and requires frequent travel. He has several important, out-of-town meetings on his schedule, and he is embarrassed about the visibility of his condition. He wants to know the cause of his skin reaction and what he can do to clear it up.

   _____

   _____

   _____

3. Meredith, a 27-year-old graphic designer, has come in for her annual wellness exam. About six months ago, she began to regularly visit a tanning salon because she thinks her skin is "pasty" and she wants to "look healthy." Over the summer, she limited her use of sunscreen and protective clothing to capitalize on tanning season. Meredith is light skinned, and her 32-year-old sister was recently diagnosed with skin cancer. She wants to minimize her own risks for developing skin cancer.

   _____

   _____

   _____

4. Florence is a 21-year-old college student. For more than a year, she has wanted to get a tattoo. One evening, on her way back to her dormitory from a physics class, Florence stops by Bob's Tattoo & Piercing Emporium on the spur of the moment. The facility appears to be a bit unsanitary, but Florence proceeds with her decision to get a small tattoo of her favorite musical instrument, the violin, in a discreet location on her left ankle. Within a week she develops redness, pain, and swelling at the tattoo site.

   _____

   _____

   _____

Lesson 8.3

Key Terms Review

Multiple Choice: *Write the letter that corresponds to the correct answer in the blank space.*

_____ 1. The teeth consist of _____ distinct parts.
- A. three
- B. four
- C. five
- D. seven

_____ 2. What is the term for the visible portion of the tooth?
- A. crown
- B. neck
- C. enamel
- D. pulp cavity

_____ 3. What is the term for the hard, white substance made of calcium that protects the crown of the tooth?
- A. dentin
- B. enamel
- C. neck
- D. pulp cavity

_____ 4. What is the term for the deepest layer of the tooth?
- A. bone
- B. dentin
- C. pulp cavity
- D. root

_____ 5. What is the name for the four teeth at the front of the mouth on the upper and lower jaws?
- A. canines
- B. premolars
- C. incisors
- D. bicuspids

_____ 6. What is the term for the sticky, colorless film that coats the teeth and dissolves their protective enamel surfaces?
- A. dentin
- B. cavity
- C. tartar
- D. plaque

_____ 7. What is another term for *cavities*?
- A. periodontitis
- B. gingivitis
- C. dental caries
- D. none of the above

_____ 8. When plaque is not removed from the teeth, it mixes with minerals to become a hard substance known as _____.
- A. periodontitis
- B. dentin
- C. enamel
- D. tartar

_____ 9. What is the medical term for inflammation of the gums?
- A. gingivitis
- B. gingidontitis
- C. periogingivitis
- D. dentitis

_____ 10. What disease is the result of bacterial infection beneath the gum tissue that destroys the gums and bone?
- A. periodontitis
- B. dental caries
- C. enamel erosion
- D. bruxism

Matching: *Match each definition to its term by writing the letter corresponding to the term in the blank space.*

_____ 11. Objects close to the eye appear clear, while objects farther away appear blurry.

_____ 12. The lens of the eye loses its elasticity, making it harder to see objects that are close.

_____ 13. Light focuses behind the retina instead of on the retina; as a result, distant objects are seen more clearly than nearby objects.

_____ 14. The eye does not focus light evenly onto the retina, resulting in blurred vision.

- A. myopia
- B. hyperopia
- C. astigmatism
- D. presbyopia

Lesson 8.3

Finding Reliable Health Information

For this activity, you will find three sources of reliable information for each of the three topics listed below. You may use the sources of information given in Figure 1.6, "Health and Safety Information," or you may research your own sources. For each source, write the name of the organization and the title of the article or web page. If the source does not appear in Figure 1.6, list its website address as well. Do not use a source more than once.

Topic: *Gingivitis*

1. A. Website #1 (name of organization) _____
   B. Title of article or web page _____
2. A. Website #2 (name of organization) _____
   B. Title of article or web page _____
3. A. Website #3 (name of organization) _____
   B. Title of article or web page _____

Topic: *Myopia*

1. A. Website #1 (name of organization) _____
   B. Title of article or web page _____
2. A. Website #2 (name of organization) _____
   B. Title of article or web page _____
3. A. Website #3 (name of organization) _____
   B. Title of article or web page _____

Topic: *Hearing loss*

1. A. Website #1 (name of organization) _____
   B. Title of article or web page _____
2. A. Website #2 (name of organization) _____
   B. Title of article or web page _____
3. A. Website #3 (name of organization) _____
   B. Title of article or web page _____

After compiling the above information about your sources, answer the following questions:

1. Of the three sources you chose for each topic, which sources were most reliable? How do you know?

   _____

   _____

2. Which sources provided the most interesting information? Write three facts you learned about each topic.

   _____

   _____

Chapter 8

Reading Practice

Reread the following passage from the textbook. Then answer the questions that follow.

Common Hearing Problems

The most serious health problem associated with the ears is permanent loss of hearing. Hearing loss is typically caused by damage to the inner ear. This damage is often the result of repeated exposure to excessively loud sounds, which can cause damage to the nerve cells in the cochlea. This may mean exposure to loud music through headphones. One recent study found that 12.5% of children and teenagers (6 to 19 years of age) experience hearing loss caused by using headphones or ear buds at too high a volume.

Sound intensity, or loudness, is measured in units called *decibels*. You can experience hearing loss by listening to sounds at or above 85 decibels over an extended period of time. The louder the sound, the less time it takes for hearing damage to occur.

Hearing loss can also be caused more suddenly by a ruptured eardrum. This can be caused by loud blasts of noise, sudden changes in pressure, insertion of an object into the ear, or an infection. In fact, just one exposure to a very loud sound, blast, or impulse (at or above 120 decibels) can cause hearing loss.

Unfortunately, many people do not notice that they are losing their hearing because damage from noise exposure is usually gradual. By the time they notice, they have substantial symptoms of permanent hearing loss. Early signs of hearing damage include

- difficulty hearing relatively soft sounds, such as doorbells;
- difficulty understanding speech during telephone conversations or in noisy environments;
- and pain or ringing in the ears, or *tinnitus*, after exposure to excessively loud sounds.

Protecting Your Hearing

Once hearing is lost, it cannot be completely brought back. It is important, therefore, to protect your ears. There are several simple ways to do so. Avoid exposure to very high levels of noise, such as at rock concerts, dances, or construction sites, whenever possible. You should also avoid listening to music at high volume levels (above 85 decibels), especially when using headphones.

_____ 1. What is the author's main idea in this passage?

    A. Permanent hearing loss is the most serious health problem associated with the ears.

    B. Hearing loss is often the result of repeated exposure to excessively loud sounds.

    C. Once hearing is lost, it cannot be completely brought back.

    D. According to a recent study, 12.5% of children and teenagers experience hearing loss caused by using headphones or earbuds at too high a volume.

_____ 2. Because hearing loss is irreversible, which of the following behaviors does the author recommend?

    A. protecting the ears (by wearing earplugs, for example)

    B. avoiding exposure to very high levels of noise

    C. listening to music at safe volume levels (below 85 decibels), especially when using headphones

    D. all of the above

_____ 3. What is the definition of *tinnitus*?

    A. inability to understand speech in a noisy environment

    B. muffled hearing

    C. ringing in the ears

    D. sharp pain in the ears

Chapter 8

Practice Test

Completion: *Write the term that completes the statement in the space provided.*

1. The outer layer of the skin is called the _____.

2. The _____ contains hair follicles that hold the hair roots.

3. The skin consists of water, protein, lipids, and _____.

4. The skin _____ the internal organs, muscles, bones, ligaments, and other structures and tissues in the body.

5. _____ determine what your hair looks like—whether it is curly, straight, thick, or thin.

6. _____ is another term for eczema, a chronic disease characterized by red, swollen, itchy, dry patches of skin.

7. Eczema is a _____ disease; this means that it recurs over time.

8. Most skin cancers are caused by exposure to _____.

9. _____ is a sticky, colorless film that coats the teeth and dissolves their protective enamel surfaces.

10. Inflammation of the gums is called _____.

True/False: *Indicate whether each statement below is true or false by circling either T or F.*

T F 11. In the eye, nerve impulses travel from the brain to the retina via the optic nerve.

T F 12. Vision problems are more common in older people because aging can cause changes in parts of the eye.

T F 13. The pupil is the part of the eye that influences how much light can enter the inner eye.

T F 14. Hyperopia is a condition in which objects close to the eye appear blurry, while objects farther away appear clear.

T F 15. The cochlea is the part of the middle ear that vibrates in response to sound.

Multiple Choice: *Write the letter that corresponds to the correct answer in the blank space.*

_____ 16. The innermost layer of skin, which contains fat, blood vessels, and nerve endings, is called the _____.

    A. epidermis   C. hypodermis

    B. dermis   D. sebaceous gland

_____ 17. Collagen and _____ are two proteins that provide support and elasticity to the skin.

    A. elastin   C. melanin

    B. sebum   D. lipids

_____ 18. The pointy teeth situated beside the incisors in your mouth are called _____.

    A. bicuspids   C. premolars

    B. canines   D. wisdom teeth

_____ 19. Repeated clenching and grinding of the teeth is called _____.

    A. bruxism   C. presbyopia

    B. misalignment   D. tinnitus

_____ 20. The _____ is a spiral tube in the inner ear that senses sound vibrations and transmits them to the auditory nerve.

    A. eardrum   C. cochlea

    B. pinna   D. semicircular canal

Matching: *Match each key term to its definition by writing the letter of the term in the space provided.*

_____ 21. invisible type of radiation that comes from the sun, tanning beds, and sunlamps

_____ 22. product that stops or dries up perspiration

_____ 23. the clear tissue that covers the front of the eye

_____ 24. infection caused by bacteria getting under the gum tissue and destroying the gums and bone

_____ 25. condition in which the eye does not focus light evenly onto the retina, causing objects to appear blurry

_____ 26. medical doctor who specializes in skin care

_____ 27. the units by which sound intensity, or loudness, is measured

_____ 28. the innermost, light-sensitive area of the eye; composed of photoreceptors that convert light into nerve impulses and electrical signals

_____ 29. term meaning "tooth decay"

_____ 30. the colored part of the eye

A. antiperspirant

B. astigmatism

C. dermatologist

D. ultraviolet (UV) light

E. dental caries

F. periodontitis

G. iris

H. cornea

I. retina

J. decibels

Short Answer: *On a separate sheet of paper, answer the following questions using what you have learned in this chapter.*

31. Describe the major functions of the skin.

32. Describe the ways in which you can prevent hearing loss.

Lesson 9.1

Key Terms Review

Multiple Choice: *Write the letter that corresponds to the correct answer in the blank space.*

_____ 1. Which of the following is *not* a form of smokeless tobacco?

    A. cigars   C. chewing tobacco

    B. snuff   D. dissolvable tobacco

_____ 2. Substances that cause cancer are called _____.

    A. tar   C. carbohydrates

    B. pathogens   D. carcinogens

_____ 3. The substance that gives tobacco products their addictive quality is _____.

    A. carbon monoxide   C. lead

    B. nicotine   D. tar

_____ 4. Which of the following is *not* true of tobacco?

    A. Tobacco leaves are used to produce cigarettes and smokeless tobacco products.

    B. Tobacco leaves contain the chemical nicotine.

    C. Smokeless tobacco products are not associated with addiction or serious health consequences.

    D. The most common method of using tobacco is smoking cigarettes.

_____ 5. Cigarettes contain a poisonous gas called _____, which interferes with the ability of blood cells to carry oxygen.

    A. carbon monoxide   C. carcinogens

    B. lead   D. tar

_____ 6. Smokeless tobacco users can develop _____, a condition characterized by white, leathery spots inside the mouth.

    A. emphysema   C. asthma

    B. chronic bronchitis   D. leukoplakia

_____ 7. _____ is a thick, sticky residue of burning tobacco that can build up in the lungs and cause disease.

    A. Carbon monoxide   C. Tar

    B. Nicotine   D. Lead

Matching: *Match each statement about a tobacco-related lung disease with the name of the disease. Write the letter corresponding to the disease in the blank space. One term will not be used.*

_____ 8. a group of diseases that make breathing more difficult

_____ 9. disease in which abnormal cells in one or both lungs grow rapidly and form a mass or tumor

_____ 10. disease characterized by the destruction of the alveoli

_____ 11. condition characterized by swelling and irritation of the bronchial tubes

_____ 12. disease in which airflow to and from the lungs is blocked; can be triggered by inhaling smoke

    A. asthma

    B. chronic bronchitis

    C. chronic obstructive pulmonary disease (COPD)

    D. emphysema

    E. leukoplakia

    F. lung cancer

Name _____ Date _____

Smoking and Your Respiratory System

Analyzing Data: *Using the illustration of the respiratory system below, answer the following questions. If needed, you may also refer to Background Lesson 4, "Respiratory System," in your textbook.*

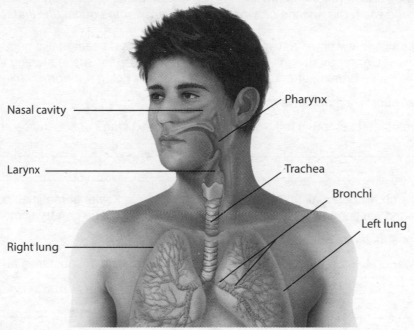

Nasal cavity

Pharynx

Larynx

Trachea

Bronchi

Left lung

Right lung

Body Scientific International, LLC

1. A. What are cilia and what role do they play in the respiratory system?

_____

   B. In what three structures are the cilia located? Circle these three structures on the above illustration.

_____

   C. How does smoking impact the functioning of cilia?

_____

2. A. What is the function of the bronchi (or bronchial tubes)?

_____

   B. How does smoking affect the functioning of bronchi?

_____

   C. Which two smoking-related diseases are characterized by swollen and irritated bronchial tubes?

_____

3. A. What are alveoli and what role do they play in the respiratory system?

_____

   B. How does smoking impact the alveoli?

_____

   C. Which smoking-related disease is characterized by destruction of the alveoli?

_____

Lesson 9.2

Identifying the Stages of Substance Abuse

Each of the following scenarios describes a person who is abusing a substance. For each scenario, determine which stage of substance abuse (experimentation, regular use, tolerance, or dependence and addiction) is described. Write your answer in the spaces provided and then answer the questions that follow.

1. Celeste used to smoke a few times a week, and for a long time that seemed like enough. However, Celeste notices that a pack of cigarettes doesn't last her as long as it used to. She is starting to smoke before classes, during her lunch breaks, after her last class, and when doing her homework in the evenings.

   A. Which stage of substance abuse is this? _____

   B. What can Celeste do to stop herself from moving to the next stage of substance abuse?

   _____

   _____

2. Xavier is a catcher on his baseball team, and at baseball games, Xavier sometimes sees some players chewing tobacco and spitting in the dugout. He is curious and asks if he can try some.

   A. Which stage of substance abuse is this?_____

   B. What can Xavier do to stop himself from moving to the next stage of substance abuse?

   _____

   _____

3. Justin smokes when he feels stressed-out, usually following an argument with his parents or after a particularly difficult day at school. He feels that smoking relaxes him. Lately, however, he's noticed that he needs to smoke two cigarettes to get the same relaxed feeling he used to get after only one.

   A. Which stage of substance abuse is this?_____

   B. What circumstances trigger Justin's desire to smoke?

   _____

   C. What can Justin do to stop himself from moving to the next stage of substance abuse?

   _____

   _____

   D. Describe two healthy strategies Justin can use to cope with the circumstances that trigger his desire to smoke.

   _____

   _____

4. After smoking regularly for a year, Hannah decides to quit. But going without cigarettes is harder than she thought. After only a few days, she feels jittery, irritable, and sick to her stomach. She experiences frequent and intense cravings for cigarettes. She is afraid that she will never feel like her "normal" self without them.

   A. Which stage of substance abuse is this?_____

   B. Describe three healthy strategies Hannah can use to help herself quit smoking.

   _____

   _____

   _____

Can This Friendship Be Saved?

Asia and Lena have been best friends since third grade. Now they are both in the tenth grade and go to the same high school. Lena recently began smoking. Asia does not smoke and does not like to be around cigarette smoke. Lena's smoking has led to tension in their relationship. For each of the following situations, describe what you think Asia should do. Then summarize the impact of Lena's smoking on Asia and their relationship. After assessing all of these situations, explain why you think Asia and Lena's friendship can or cannot be saved.

1. In the morning, Asia picks up Lena at her house and gives her a ride to school. Lena lights up a cigarette in the car. Asia doesn't like the way the smoke makes her car, clothes, and hair smell. She knows that breathing secondhand smoke can affect her health. What should Asia say or do?

   _____

   _____

2. Lena and Asia used to have lunch together in the cafeteria. But now that Lena smokes, she wants to go off campus during lunch breaks so she can have a cigarette. Lena hitches a ride with her new smoker friends and wants Asia to come along. What should Asia say or do?

   _____

   _____

3. Lena and Asia used to enjoy doing things together on weekends. But since Lena began smoking, she spends most of her allowance on cigarettes. When Asia suggests they go see a movie or go to the mall, Lena says she's broke. Asia misses the fun times they used to have. What should Asia say or do?

   _____

   _____

4. Lena's parents don't know that she smokes. Lena says that if they knew, she would be "grounded for life." One day, Asia goes to Lena's house after school, and Lena smokes several cigarettes while they play a game. When Lena's father comes home, he asks why Asia and Lena smell like cigarettes. Lena says, "We just walked by a group of kids who were smoking—right, Asia?" Asia can get grounded by her own parents for lying. What should Asia say or do?

   _____

   _____

5. Now that she smokes, Lena is spending more and more time hanging out with other teenagers who smoke. Lena invites Asia to a party where she can meet her new friends. When Asia arrives, everyone is smoking, including Lena. "Come on, Asia, have a puff," says Lena as she tries to hand Asia a cigarette. Lena's new friends chime in, "Yeah, it won't bite you!" Asia feels all their eyes on her and she wants desperately to fit in. What should Asia say or do?

   _____

   _____

6. Based on the situations above, summarize how Lena's smoking is impacting Asia and their friendship. Do you think the girls can or should remain best friends? Why or why not?

   _____

   _____

Lesson 9.3

You Be the Government

For this activity, imagine that you are the elected leader of a small democratic country. You plan to improve education, clean up polluted waterways, and improve food production and safety. Your programs will cost millions of dollars that your country does not have because so much money is being spent on healthcare. Your public health secretary tells you that healthcare costs are high because about half of the population uses tobacco products, especially cigarettes. Each year, several million people die from smoking-related causes, and millions more receive healthcare for serious diseases caused by smoking or breathing secondhand smoke. Even though your government has limited control over private businesses, you decide your government must do all it can to eliminate tobacco use. For each question below, describe what you and your administration can realistically do to solve the problem.

1. What laws and regulations can your government implement to limit the marketing and advertising of tobacco products?

   _____
   _____
   _____

2. What laws and regulations can your government implement to limit the sale of tobacco products?

   _____
   _____
   _____

3. What can your government do to limit the public's exposure to secondhand smoke?

   _____
   _____
   _____

4. What can your government do to educate the public about the dangers of smoking and tobacco use?

   _____
   _____
   _____

5. What can your government do to help people addicted to tobacco products quit?

   _____
   _____
   _____

6. What laws and regulations can your government implement to regulate the price of tobacco products?

   _____
   _____
   _____

Lesson 9.3

Create an Antismoking Advertisement

In small groups, create an antismoking advertisement to convince people to stop smoking or to never begin smoking. Follow the instructions below to get started. Then create your advertisement, using the medium of your choice, and share it with the class.

Choose a target group.

Advertisements are crafted to appeal to a particular audience. Which group(s) of people will your antismoking advertisement target? Some target audiences might be teenagers, adults, women or men, people of a particular economic or ethnic group, or people who do or do not smoke. Describe your target audience below:

_____

_____

_____

_____

Choose a focus.

Choose an antismoking message you want to communicate. "Smoking is bad" is too broad. You should choose a narrower focus. For example, you might focus on the financial costs of smoking, or the fact that smoking can cause diseases and premature death. Consider what kind of antismoking message will appeal to the group you have chosen. Summarize the message of your ad in one or two sentences below:

_____

_____

_____

_____

Choose a medium for your message.

Choose a medium for you advertisement. Your group might create a flyer, a poster, a video, a podcast, or a website. When choosing your medium, consider which medium will best reach your target audience. Describe which medium your group chose and why you chose it below:

_____

_____

_____

_____

Chapter 9

Reading Practice

Reread the following passage from the textbook. Then answer the questions that follow.

The Impact of Secondhand Smoke

Secondhand smoke refers to the tobacco smoke you are exposed to in the environment. People who are regularly exposed to secondhand smoke because they live or socialize with smokers are at greater risk of developing lung cancer or heart disease.

Concerns about the dangerous effects of secondhand smoke on health have led a number of states to pass laws banning smoking in many public areas to protect the health of customers and staff. Secondhand smoke greatly affects certain population groups, including pregnant women, infants, and children.

Pregnant Women and Infants

Exposure to nicotine is particularly hazardous to a developing fetus. When a pregnant woman smokes, the nicotine and carbon monoxide she takes into her body pass through the placenta to the fetus. The immediate impact on the fetus is an increased heart rate and reduction in the amount of oxygen the fetus receives.

Women who smoke while pregnant increase their risk of miscarriage, and of having babies born prematurely or with low birth weight. Babies born to mothers who smoked or breathed secondhand smoke during pregnancy also have a higher risk factor for sudden infant death syndrome (SIDS). SIDS is the unexpected and sudden death of a baby less than one year after birth.

Children

Exposure to secondhand smoke is a major cause of health problems in children. Children exposed to second-hand smoke are more likely to have respiratory problems such as pneumonia, bronchitis, and asthma attacks. Children whose parents smoke also have higher rates of sore throats and ear infections.

Behavior-related issues common in children of mothers who smoked during pregnancy include attention deficit disorders, hyperactivity, and aggression.

_____ 1. Why have states passed laws banning smoking in public areas?

    A. They are concerned about the dangerous effects of secondhand smoke on health.

    B. They want to protect the health of customers and staff.

    C. They want to protect the health of certain population groups.

    D. all of the above

_____ 2. Which of the following statements explains how exposure to nicotine affects a developing fetus?

    A. Children exposed to secondhand smoke are more likely to have respiratory problems.

    B. Children of smokers are more likely to develop smoking habits themselves.

    C. If a pregnant woman inhales tobacco smoke, the nicotine and carbon monoxide will pass through the placenta to her fetus.

    D. none of the above

_____ 3. Which statement best expresses the main idea of this passage?

    A. Breathing secondhand smoke affects a child's physical health.

    B. Breathing secondhand smoke affects a pregnant woman's health.

    C. Breathing secondhand smoke is dangerous, especially for pregnant women, infants, and children.

    D. The government should protect people from exposure to secondhand smoke.

Chapter 9

Practice Test

Completion: *Write the term that completes the statement in the space provided.*

1. Carbon monoxide in cigarette smoke interferes with the ability of blood cells to carry _____.

2. People who smoke for at least 10 years show more _____ in their skin.

3. Smokers have _____ rates of cancer than nonsmokers.

4. _____ is finely cut or powdered tobacco that is inhaled or placed between the cheek and gum.

5. The Food and Drug Administration opposes the use of electronic cigarettes by teenagers because they can cause addiction to _____.

True/False: *Indicate whether each statement below is true or false by circling either T or F.*

T   F   6. Smoking is the leading cause of preventable death in the United States.

T   F   7. A psychological dependence occurs when the body relies on having a certain amount of a substance to function "normally."

T   F   8. Substance abuse begins with experimentation.

T   F   9. Tolerance develops when the body needs less and less of a substance to experience the effects it felt when a greater amount was used.

T   F   10. Tobacco smoke contains over 70 carcinogens.

Multiple Choice: *Write the letter that corresponds to the correct answer in the blank space.*

_____ 11. Which body system includes the heart and blood vessels?
   A. immune system
   B. respiratory system
   C. cardiovascular system
   D. nervous system

_____ 12. Which fatty substance can build up in the arteries and disrupt the flow of blood through the body?
   A. tar
   B. cilia
   C. proteins
   D. cholesterol

_____ 13. A laryngectomy is performed on people, often smokers, who have _____.
   A. cancer of the larynx
   B. lung cancer
   C. heart disease
   D. oral cancer

_____ 14. Smokers are at greater risk of becoming ill from germs that cause colds and the flu due to a weakened _____.
   A. respiratory system
   B. immune system
   C. heart
   D. lung capacity

_____ 15. In some people, inhaling cigarette smoke can irritate the lining of the airways and trigger a(n) _____.
   A. asthma attack
   B. stroke
   C. cold or flu
   D. gum disease

Name _____ Date _____

Matching: *Match each key term to its definition by writing the letter of the term in the space provided.*

_____ 16. use of a drug, or intentional misuse of prescription medication, that can cause harmful, dangerous effects

_____ 17. method of smoking cessation in which tobacco users gradually reduce their nicotine consumption

_____ 18. physical and psychological need for a substance or behavior

_____ 19. technique in which people learn to respond to stress with stress management, relaxation, and coping skills, instead of with smoking

_____ 20. unpleasant symptoms associated with an attempt to stop using a substance

_____ 21. smoking-cessation technique in which smokers avoid situations that may lead them to smoke

_____ 22. an individual's feeling that he or she must conform to the wishes of friends to earn their approval

_____ 23. condition in which a person relies on a given substance to function or feel normal

A. addiction

B. dependence

C. nicotine replacement

D. peer pressure

E. response substitution

F. stimulus control

G. substance abuse

H. withdrawal

Analyzing Data: *Use the graph below to answer the following questions.*

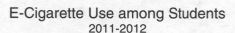

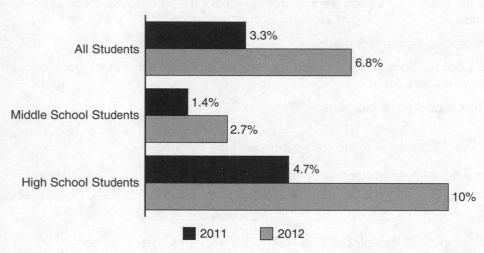

E-Cigarette Use among Students
2011-2012

All Students — 3.3% / 6.8%
Middle School Students — 1.4% / 2.7%
High School Students — 4.7% / 10%

■ 2011 ▨ 2012

Source: CDC, National Youth Tobacco Survey

24. For which group of students was e-cigarette use more popular?

_____

25. By what percentage did e-cigarette use increase between 2011 and 2012 for high school students?

_____

Short Answer: *On a separate sheet of paper, answer the following questions using what you have learned in this chapter.*

26. Compare and contrast positive and negative peer pressure, and give two examples of each.

27. Some antismoking researchers believe that the best way to prevent teenagers from smoking is to emphasize the negative effects of smoking on appearance and hygiene. Do you agree or disagree? Explain your answer.

Lesson 10.1

Alcohol and the Brain

Alcohol is a depressant, which means that it slows down the central nervous system and significantly affects the brain. Alcohol affects different parts of the brain in different ways; it disrupts physical functioning in some parts and causes psychological changes in others.

On the brain diagram below, identify each unlabeled part of the brain. Then, explain the effect that alcohol has on that part of the brain. Finally, describe a physical or psychological consequence associated with impaired function of that part. For question 1, explain the effect of alcohol on and the consequences of impairment for neurotransmitters, *which are chemicals in the brain.*

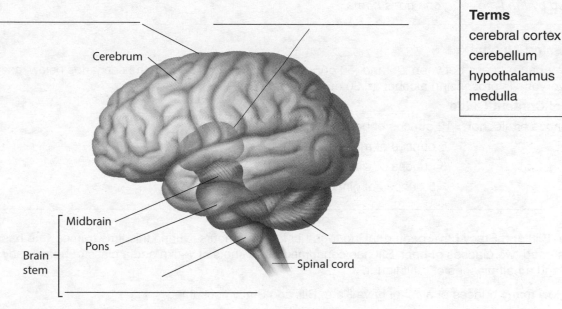

Terms
cerebral cortex
cerebellum
hypothalamus
medulla

Cerebrum

Midbrain

Pons

Brain stem

Spinal cord

1. Part of the brain: *neurotransmitters*

   Effect of alcohol: _____

   Consequences of impairment: _____

2. Part of the brain: *cerebral cortex*

   Effect of alcohol: _____

   Consequences of impairment: _____

3. Part of the brain: *cerebellum*

   Effect of alcohol: _____

   Consequences of impairment: _____

4. Part of the brain: *hypothalamus*

   Effect of alcohol: _____

   Consequences of impairment: _____

5. Part of the brain: *medulla*

   Effect of alcohol: _____

   Consequences of impairment: _____

Lesson 10.1

Level of Intoxication

Once alcohol is consumed, it stays in the body until the liver can metabolize it, or break it down. Generally, the liver can process between .25 and .50 ounces of alcohol every hour. When someone drinks a large amount of alcohol in a short period of time, also known as binge drinking, the body cannot break down the alcohol fast enough. Binge drinking results in a high blood alcohol concentration and a high level of intoxication.

Study the information in the box below about how much alcohol is in each type of drink. Then, use this information to answer the questions below. For each scenario presented, determine how many ounces of alcohol each person consumed, how much of that alcohol each person has processed, and who is the most intoxicated by the time everyone goes home.

Processing Alcohol

The liver can process between .25 and .50 ounces of alcohol each hour. In the scenarios below, assume that everyone is processing alcohol at .30 ounces per hour.

Alcohol Content Guide

0.6 ounces of alcohol = 12 ounces of beer

8 ounces of malt liquor

5 ounces of wine

1.5 ounces of gin/vodka/whiskey

---

1. Kate, Bill, and Stacy have been drinking together for three hours. During this time frame, Kate has consumed two glasses of beer. Bill has consumed three shots of vodka and a glass of beer. Stacy has had one and a half glasses of malt liquor.

    A. How many ounces of alcohol have Kate, Bill, and Stacy consumed?

    Kate: _____

    Bill: _____

    Stacy: _____

    B. How many ounces of alcohol do they process in three hours? _____

    C. How many ounces of alcohol are left unprocessed?

    Kate: _____

    Bill: _____

    Stacy: _____

    D. Who is the most intoxicated? _____

2. Gene and John arrived at the bar two hours ago. Within this time period, Gene drank two shots of vodka and a glass of malt liquor. John had one beer.

    A. How many ounces of alcohol have Gene and John consumed?

    Gene: _____

    John: _____

B. How many ounces of alcohol do they process in two hours? _____

C. How many ounces of alcohol are left unprocessed?

Gene: _____

John: _____

D. Who is the most intoxicated? _____

3. Wine is being served at this week's book discussion hour. In that hour, Lauren has consumed three glasses of wine, Andrea has had one glass, and Luke has had half a glass.

A. How many ounces of alcohol have Lauren, Andrea, and Luke consumed?

Lauren: _____

Andrea: _____

Luke: _____

B. How many ounces of alcohol do they process in one hour? _____

C. How many ounces of alcohol are left unprocessed?

Lauren: _____

Andrea: _____

Luke: _____

D. Who is the most intoxicated? _____

4. Barry is at a bachelor party for his friend Derek. During the past six hours of partying, Barry has consumed three beers and two shots of vodka. Derek has had six beers and four shots of vodka.

A. How many ounces of alcohol have Barry and Derek consumed?

Barry: _____

Derek: _____

B. How many ounces of alcohol do they process in six hours? _____

C. How many ounces of alcohol are left unprocessed?

Barry: _____

Derek: _____

D. Who is the most intoxicated? _____

Lesson 10.2

The Voice of Reason

The impaired judgment that comes with being intoxicated can cause situations that result in violence or serious injury. Just as people who know they will be drinking elect a "designated driver," imagine that you have been elected a designated "voice of reason" in each of the scenarios below. As the voice of reason, your job is to speak out to stop situations from getting out of hand and to keep your friends safe. For each of the scenarios below, describe how you would act as your friends' designated voice of reason.

1. You are hanging out at your friend Bill's house on a Friday evening. Bill has been drinking, but you have not. All night, Bill has been lamenting his poor grades and has been expressing worry that he won't be able to graduate. As he continues to drink, Bill gets more and more depressed and even mentions thoughts of suicide. You are his "voice of reason." What would you do or say?

   _____

   _____

   _____

2. You and your friend Jenny have been watching movies all night and it is now very late. Jenny has been drinking, but you have not. Jenny's family has a pool in their backyard. In the middle of one of your movies, Jenny announces that she'd like to go swimming. Jenny sneaks outside to the pool and you follow her. You know that swimming can be a dangerous activity if someone is intoxicated and not in full control of his or her actions. You are Jenny's "voice of reason." What would you do or say?

   _____

   _____

   _____

3. You and a few friends are hanging out in Jared's backyard and have started a bonfire. Although most of the people there are drinking, you and a few friends are not. Everyone seems to be having fun at first, but then you hear someone shout angrily. Before you know it, two of your friends who were drinking are shouting at each other and squaring off as though they are going to fight. You are their "voice of reason." What would you do or say?

   _____

   _____

   _____

4. You are hanging out with a few friends who are drinking casually, but you have chosen not to drink. Everyone is having a nice evening, but you begin to notice that your friend Beth is drinking more than anyone else. By the end of the evening, Beth has passed out on the couch and has already vomited once. You are worried that Beth may have alcohol poisoning, but no one else seems concerned. You are the "voice of reason." What would you do or say?

   _____

   _____

   _____

Lesson 10.2

The Effects of Underage Drinking

Although it is illegal in all states for people younger than 21 years of age to drink, underage drinkers account for 11% of all alcohol consumed in the United States. Teenagers who drink put themselves at risk for long-term health problems. They also put themselves at risk for immediate problems that can affect their health, futures, and relationships.

For each of the scenarios presented here, determine whether the teen's drinking is affecting his or her physical health, education, social life, or future.

1. Samantha's sister is annoyed with her because her drinking has gotten in the way of their old movie night tradition. Samantha has been missing more and more movie nights since she started hanging out with a new group of friends and began drinking.

   _____

   _____

2. Ben was pulled over while driving under the influence of alcohol and was charged with a DUI. As a result, he had his license suspended. Not being able to drive in the evenings means that he can't get to his part-time job at a local fast-food restaurant. He has been saving up money for college, but now he may lose his job.

   _____

   _____

3. Devon started hanging out with a new group of friends, and now he often spends his evenings drinking with them. As a result, he has missed several football practices. The season just began, and his coach cannot afford to have a player who doesn't pull his weight. Devon is cut from the team.

   _____

   _____

4. Kiki's habit of having a few drinks on the weekends with her friends has gotten out of hand. Now she's been drinking on school nights, and the hangovers she has in the mornings make it hard to concentrate in class. Recently, she failed an important test in her math class.

   _____

   _____

5. Seth spent a Saturday drinking with his friends and he knew he was too intoxicated to drive home. Instead, he walked home, but the weather was very cold that evening. As a result, Seth caught a bad cold and had to stay in bed for several days.

   _____

   _____

Lesson 10.3

Nature or Nurture?

A person's biology, genes, and environment impact whether he or she abuses or even uses alcohol. For example, an adopted child with an alcoholic biological parent is four times more likely to become a problem drinker than an adopted child whose biological parents are not alcoholics. Similarly, environment can impact whether a person drinks. Someone whose caregivers or friends drink alcohol is more likely to drink than someone whose caregivers and friends do not drink alcohol. In each of the following scenarios, determine which factor—nature (genes) or nurture (environment)—is influencing a person's alcohol use and identify two ways the person can avoid the pressure and temptation to drink alcohol.

1. Becky has grown up surrounded by alcohol at family gatherings during the holidays. When she begins celebrating the holidays—or any occasion—on her own, she also includes alcohol in the festivities.

   _____

   _____

   _____

2. When Jared was growing up, his biological father used to yell and become irrationally angry. Many years later, Jared's older brother explained that this was because their father was an alcoholic. Jared notices that when he drinks, he often yells and becomes angry as well.

   _____

   _____

   _____

3. Leslie was never interested in drinking when she was growing up and there wasn't much alcohol in her home. When she started high school, however, Leslie began hanging out with a new group of friends who drank more often. Soon, Leslie began drinking regularly with her friends.

   _____

   _____

   _____

4. Carol and Caryn are twins. When the girls were in high school, Carol often spent her weekends drinking with friends, sometimes to the point of abusing alcohol. Later, when the twins went to college, Caryn began drinking and abusing alcohol as well.

   _____

   _____

   _____

5. Neither of Liam's parents drink, and none of his older siblings drink either. However, Liam enjoys watching movies about gangsters from the 1920s who are often shown drinking on screen. Liam starts drinking here and there with some friends and then becomes a binge drinker.

   _____

   _____

   _____

Lesson 10.3

Alcohol Ad Analysis

Even though you might think you're ignoring the ads on TV, they can still be persuasive and influence people's behavior. Ads for alcohol are particularly dangerous because they do not show the harmful consequences associated with drinking. Often, ads for alcohol focus instead on how attractive or popular drinking can supposedly make you.

During one evening of watching TV, track the ads that you see. Using the chart below, record what each ad was for, the message or focus of each ad, and whether the ad was presented during teen programming. Then, answer the questions below.

Product	Message/Focus	Program

1. How many ads for alcohol did you see? How many were positive?

   _____

   _____

2. What were the main messages of these alcohol ads?

   _____

   _____

3. If teenagers saw these ads without knowing anything else about alcohol, what would they think about drinking alcohol?

   _____

   _____

4. Do you think that making ads more realistic or changing the times at which alcohol ads run would help decrease amounts of teen drinking? Why or why not?

   _____

   _____

   _____

Lesson 10.4

Using Refusal Skills

The best way to protect yourself from the consequences of alcohol use is to never begin drinking. This can be difficult if friends are pressuring you to try alcohol, but you can develop and practice refusal skills to resist peer pressure. Refusal skills are your ability to stand up to pressures and influences that hinder your progress toward wellness. Often, refusal skills include saying "no," explaining why you have made your choice, or even leaving the situation completely.

For each of the following scenarios, explain what you might say to refuse your friend's offer of alcohol. Keep in mind that you may need to leave the situation to avoid further peer pressure. Try to be creative and specific with your responses.

1. On Saturday evening, you are invited to a party at your friend's house. Even though you know you have some homework to do, you decide to go to the party for a few hours. When you arrive, you realize that there are no adults present at the party and that several people have brought alcohol. You are already uncomfortable with the situation when your best friend offers you a drink.

   _____

   _____

2. You and a group of friends are hanging out on a Wednesday night. Halfway through the evening, some of your friends decide to start drinking. You know that it's a school night, you have a test first thing in the morning, and you have to leave soon anyway. You're about to leave when your friend offers you a drink and begs you to stay.

   _____

   _____

3. On the Friday afternoon before summer vacation starts, you notice invitations to a party being handed out. One of these invitations is slipped into your locker. When you see who is throwing the party, you know that there will be alcohol there. You have made the choice not to drink and you know that people at the party will try to pressure you into drinking.

   _____

   _____

4. You and your friends are holding a game night, and the night is going well. Everyone is having fun, and you're enjoying just hanging out with your friends and playing games. A friend you don't know very well wants to make the next game into a drinking game. Everyone else agrees with this person and seems to like the idea. Your friends tell you, "it'll be fun," but you were already having fun without alcohol.

   _____

   _____

5. You are at a weekend party where alcohol is being served. So far, you've found it easy to refuse your friends' offers of alcohol. Then you notice that the boy or girl you have a crush on is also drinking. You really want to impress this person and you want this person to like you, but you also don't want to drink. Your crush offers to get you a drink. What do you say?

   _____

   _____

Chapter 10

Reading Practice

Reread the following passage from the textbook. Then answer the questions that follow.

Alcoholism

In contrast to problem drinkers, people who are **alcoholics** are both psychologically and physically addicted to alcohol. **Alcoholism**, or complete dependency on alcohol, is recognized as a disease by the Centers for Disease Control and Prevention (CDC). Physical addiction to alcohol occurs when a person needs to consume alcohol so he or she can function "normally."

People do not suddenly become alcoholics. Instead, people generally follow the stages of substance abuse, which you learned about in Chapter 9. The first stage of substance abuse is *experimentation*. Experimentation with alcohol can lead to the second stage of substance abuse, *regular use*. Some people may stop at this stage.

People who become alcoholics, however, enter the third stage of substance abuse—*tolerance*. Gradually, the user consumes larger amounts of alcohol to feel the same effects. The tolerance stage of alcohol abuse resembles problem drinking.

The final stage of substance abuse, *dependence and addiction*, occurs when the user is psychologically and physically dependent on alcohol. Some health professionals refer to this as *late-stage alcoholism*.

1. _____ is recognized as a disease by the Centers for Disease Control and Prevention.
    - A. Tolerance
    - B. Experimentation
    - C. Regular use
    - D. Alcoholism

2. Which of the following is *not* a stage of substance abuse?
    - A. tolerance
    - B. quitting
    - C. dependence and addiction
    - D. experimentation

3. The tolerance stage of alcohol abuse resembles _____.
    - A. problem drinking
    - B. moderate drinking
    - C. alcoholism
    - D. late-stage alcoholism

4. The final stage of substance abuse is sometimes referred to as _____.
    - A. moderate drinking
    - B. social drinking
    - C. late-stage alcoholism
    - D. problem drinking

Chapter 10

Practice Test

Completion: *Write the term that completes the statement in the space provided.*

1. The word _____ is a general term used to describe a drink that contains a certain amount of ethanol.

2. The psychological restraint that discourages people from engaging in dangerous behaviors is known as _____.

3. The condition known as _____ is a buildup of scar tissue in the liver.

4. The term _____ describes the consumption of enough alcohol that a person experiences problems in his or her daily life.

5. One of the first steps in recovery for all alcoholics is a "drying out" process known as _____.

True/False: *Indicate whether each statement below is true or false by circling either T or F.*

T   F   6. When alcohol reaches the brain, it does *not* affect neurotransmitters.

T   F   7. Alcohol use can cause strained relationships among family and friends.

T   F   8. People who have been drinking are less likely to behave violently than people who have not been drinking.

T   F   9. Moderate drinking is also known as *social drinking*.

T   F   10. Many studies show that most teenagers do not actually drink.

Multiple Choice: *Write the letter that corresponds to the correct answer in the blank space.*

_____ 11. Alcohol disrupts functioning of the _____, which controls movement and balance.
   A. medulla
   B. cerebellum
   C. cerebral cortex
   D. pituitary gland

_____ 12. Which of the following is *not* a symptom of alcohol poisoning?
   A. mental confusion
   B. vomiting
   C. hair loss
   D. hypothermia

_____ 13. Another term for complete dependency on alcohol is _____.
   A. alcoholism
   B. moderate drinking
   C. tolerance
   D. social drinking

_____ 14. Which of the following is *not* an environmental factor for alcohol use?
   A. alcohol at family parties
   B. an alcoholic, biological parent
   C. peer pressure from friends
   D. TV and movies that include alcohol use

_____ 15. Self-management techniques for people with drinking problems do *not* include_____.
   A. avoiding situations where alcohol is present
   B. developing strategies for refusing alcohol
   C. engaging in social drinking
   D. learning new strategies for managing stress

Name _____

Matching: *Match each key term to its definition by writing the letter of the term in the space provided.*

_____ 16. term for the uncomfortable physical symptoms caused by excessive alcohol consumption

_____ 17. a legal offense that occurs when a person has driven with a blood alcohol concentration over 0.08

_____ 18. term for a group of serious physical and mental birth defects caused by a woman's consumption of alcohol while pregnant

_____ 19. a medical emergency that occurs when a high blood alcohol concentration suppresses the central nervous system

_____ 20. a substance that slows the central nervous system and causes chemical changes in the brain

_____ 21. a disease in which a person is completely dependent on alcohol

_____ 22. the consumption of a large amount of alcohol in a short period of time

_____ 23. encouraging an addict's destructive behaviors, either intentionally or unintentionally

A. depressant

B. alcohol poisoning

C. alcoholism

D. binge drinking

E. enabling

F. driving under the influence (DUI)

G. hangover

H. fetal alcohol syndrome (FAS)

Analyzing Data: *The graph below shows the percentage of high school seniors who reported having five or more drinks in a row in the past two weeks. The data is separated by gender, and the graph describes which types of drinks the high school students reported having. Study the data in this graph and then answer the questions that follow. For the purposes of this practice test, assume the study surveyed 13,000 high school seniors.*

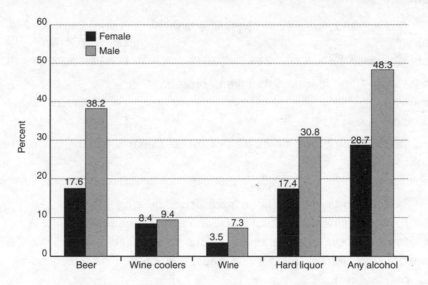

Source: Bachman et al. (2001).

24. How many more males than females had five or more drinks of any alcohol? _____

25. What percentage of teens—males and females—had five or more drinks of any alcohol? _____

26. Generally, who has five or more drinks of alcohol in a row more often—males or females? Why do you think this is the case?

_____

Short Answer: *On a separate sheet of paper, answer the following questions using what you have learned in this chapter.*

27. What do you think is the most persuasive argument that could be used to get teens to stop drinking?

28. If you see a friend or family member abusing alcohol, what is the best thing you can do to help him or her?

Name _____ Date _____

Key Concepts Review

Multiple Choice: *Write the letter that corresponds to the correct answer in the blank space.*

_____ 1. Which of the following are main reasons that people use medications?
  A. to treat symptoms of an illness   C. to cure a disease
  B. to manage a disease   D. all of the above

_____ 2. Which type of drug kills or slows the growth of bacteria?
  A. analgesics   C. antibiotics
  B. opiates   D. transdermal patches

_____ 3. Which type of medication works with the body's natural immune system to reduce the risk of developing an infection or disease?
  A. vaccinations   C. opiates
  B. antibiotics   D. anesthetics

_____ 4. Which of the following are methods in which medication can be taken?
  A. pills or liquids   C. inhalers
  B. topical creams, gels, or other   D. all of the above
     ointments

_____ 5. Which of the following is *not* an example of an opioid, or a drug prescribed to relieve pain?
  A. Vicodin®   C. OxyContin®
  B. acetaminophen   D. Percocet®

_____ 6. What is another name for drugs that are *depressants*?
  A. sedatives   C. tranquilizers
  B. stimulants   D. both A and C

_____ 7. Which of the following drugs increases the level of dopamine in the brain, producing euphoria?
  A. amphetamines   C. opioids
  B. barbiturates   D. antibiotics

_____ 8. Which of the following best describes *medication abuse*?
  A. not following the instructions for use of a particular medication
  B. not following proper disposal methods for prescription or over-the-counter medications
  C. intentional use of medication for any reason other than that prescribed
  D. none of the above

_____ 9. Which of the following drugs slow(s) a person's central nervous system, causing his or her rate of breathing and heart rate to decrease?
  A. anti-anxiety medications   C. barbiturates used for surgical
  B. sleep medications   procedures or seizure disorders
                                              D. all of the above

Matching: *Match each prescription medication with its common side effects when abused. Write the letter of the medication in the blank space.*

_____ 10. increased body temperature, irregular heartbeat, feelings of hostility   A. opioids
            and paranoia
                                                                                      B. depressants
_____ 11. slowed breathing rate, low blood pressure, unconsciousness, coma, and
            death (especially when combined with alcohol or other depressants)   C. stimulants

_____ 12. depression, chronic fatigue, breathing problems, difficulty sleeping,
            coma, death (often by overdose)

Lesson 11.2

Can This Friendship Be Saved?

Young stand-up comedians David and Jay quickly formed a friendship when they both joined the comedy circuit a year ago. They frequently perform their routines in comedy clubs and other venues where liquor and illicit drugs are readily available. Jay avoids drugs and has never smoked a cigarette because his father died of lung cancer when Jay was young. David has recently begun to use a variety of drugs, including marijuana and cocaine. Jay is concerned that David is developing a physical addiction, but he is not sure how to help his friend without coming across as judgmental. For each of the following situations, describe what you think Jay should do. Then summarize the impact David's drug use is having on his friendship with Jay. Explain why you think their friendship can or cannot be saved.

1. Each night before David goes onstage to perform his comedy routine, he snorts cocaine. Almost instantly, he feels more energetic and mentally alert. Jay thinks that David gets "too wired" because he moves at a frenetic pace, and at times his joke delivery is so rapid that some of his words cannot be deciphered. David tells Jay that the "blow" helps him get through his late-night performances, especially when he is fatigued after working all day at his job as a production assistant at a local TV station. David says that he can "stop using any time." What should Jay say or do?

   _____

   _____

   _____

2. One night after performing, David suffers side effects that he has previously never experienced during cocaine use. His heart is beating so rapidly that he thinks he might have a heart attack. In addition, David is certain that Jimmy, a new talent on the comedy scene, has been "stealing" David's jokes. David gets into an altercation with Jimmy and accuses him of being a thief. Jay attempts to calm David down by distracting him, and tries to persuade him that they should leave the comedy club. He offers to give his friend a ride home, but David's belligerence and paranoia seem to be impenetrable. What should Jay say or do?

   _____

   _____

   _____

3. Early one evening, David drives to Jay's apartment to pick him up. They are planning to perform their comedy routines during open-mike night at a new club on the opposite side of the city. As Jay slides into the front passenger seat of David's pickup truck, he instantly recognizes the odor of marijuana. David is smoking a joint. He inhales deeply and offers the joint to Jay. "No, I'm good," Jay says, declining David's offer. Jay tells David that driving under the influence of marijuana is not only against the law, but it also affects a person's thinking, motor skills, and sensory perception. David says it doesn't do that to him. What should Jay say or do?

   _____

   _____

   _____

4. Based on the situations above, summarize the ways in which David's abuse of illegal drugs is affecting his friendship with Jay. Do you think the comedians can or should maintain a friendship? Why or why not?

   _____

   _____

   _____

Lesson 11.3

Create an Antidrug Advertisement

In small groups, create an antidrug advertisement to convince people to stop or never start abusing drugs (or using illegal drugs). Follow the instructions below to get started. Then create your advertisement, using the medium of your choice, and share it with the class. All of the advertisements created by the class will constitute an antidrug campaign.

Choose a target group.

Advertisements are created to appeal to a particular audience. Which group(s) of people will your antidrug advertisement target? Some target audiences might be teenagers, adults, women or men, people of a particular economic or ethnic group, or people who do or do not use drugs. Describe your target audience below:

_____

_____

_____

_____

Choose a focus.

Choose an antidrug message you want to communicate. "Using drugs is bad" is too broad a statement. You should choose a narrower focus. For example, you might focus on the harmful physical and psychological effects of using drugs, including the possibly fatal results, or on the negative social perceptions of drug abusers. Consider what kind of antidrug message will appeal to the group you have chosen. Summarize the message of your advertisement in one or two sentences below:

_____

_____

_____

_____

Choose a medium for your message.

Choose a medium for your advertisement. Your group might create a flyer, poster, video, podcast, or website. When choosing your medium, consider which medium will best reach your target audience. Describe which medium your group chose and why you chose it below:

_____

_____

_____

_____

Chapter 11

Reading Practice

Reread the following passage from the textbook. Then answer the questions on the next page.

Although anyone can abuse and become addicted to a drug, experts point to certain risk factors that could increase a person's chances of becoming addicted.

Biological Makeup

A person's genetic makeup influences whether he or she will become addicted to drugs. People whose parents have addiction problems are at greater risk of becoming addicts themselves. Experts believe that people's genes account for about half of their risk of becoming addicted to drugs. A person's biological makeup can also influence his or her personality. Some people have a cautious personality and are averse to risk taking. These people may be reluctant to use drugs due to their concerns about the consequences. Other people are more curious and likely to take risks. Unfortunately, a willingness to take risks and use drugs can lead to addiction.

Mental Health Problems

People who have mental health problems, such as depression or anxiety, may use drugs to cope with their symptoms. The use of drugs by an individual to treat problems and symptoms not diagnosed by a medical doctor is called *self-medication*. People who self-medicate do not get the professional help they need to successfully diagnose and treat their condition. Self-medicating also puts people at risk of developing addictions and more severe mental health problems.

Stage of Development

The earlier a person begins using a drug, the more likely he or she is to abuse and become addicted to that drug. Teenagers are at particular risk of becoming addicted to drugs. This is partly because the brains of teenagers are still developing in the areas that govern decision making, judgment, and self-control.

Environment

The environment in which people live has an impact on their potential exposure to drugs and whether they feel pressured to use drugs. Environment includes a person's neighborhood, school, family, and peers. For example, teens may feel pressured to try drugs if they attend parties where drugs are present.

A person's environment also includes social institutions, such as the media, that reflect and reinforce social values. Some research suggests that teenagers who see drug use in movies are more likely to experiment with drugs themselves. Another study found that half of high school students surveyed believed that seeing professional athletes use steroids influenced their friends' decisions to use steroids.

Choosing to live a drug-free lifestyle can be challenging for teens, especially when their environment exposes them to drugs and the pressures of trying them. There are strategies, however, that teens can use to refuse drugs.

(Continued)

Name _____

_____ 1. According to experts, genetic makeup accounts for approximately what percentage of people's risk of becoming addicted to drugs?

    A. 25%

    B. 50%

    C. 75%

    D. Genetic makeup does not factor into the risk of developing a drug addiction.

_____ 2. Which of the following statements is applicable to people who self-medicate?

    A. People who self-medicate do not get the professional help they need to successfully diagnose and treat their conditions.

    B. Self-medicating puts people at risk of developing addictions and more severe mental health problems.

    C. People who have mental health problems, such as depression or anxiety, may be prescribed drugs to cope with their symptoms.

    D. all of the above

_____ 3. Which of the following factors puts teenagers (in particular) at risk for becoming addicted to drugs?

    A. Teenagers' brains are still developing in the areas that govern decision making, judgment, and self-control.

    B. Teenagers are more likely than adults to be exposed to drugs that are addictive.

    C. Teenagers in general are more curious and adventurous.

    D. both A and C

_____ 4. A teenager's environment can influence his or her decision to use drugs. Which of the following factors contribute to a teenager's environment?

    A. family

    B. neighborhood

    C. media

    D. all of the above

_____ 5. According to a survey, approximately what percentage of high school students believe that the use of steroids by professional athletes influenced a friend's decision to use steroids?

    A. 25%

    B. 50%

    C. 65%

    D. Teenagers do not believe that steroid use is influenced to any degree by the behaviors of professional athletes.

_____ 6. Which statement best expresses the main idea of this passage?

    A. Choosing to live a drug-free lifestyle can be challenging for teens.

    B. A person's biological makeup can influence his or her risk of developing a drug addiction.

    C. Although anyone can abuse and become addicted to a drug, certain risk factors could increase a person's chances of becoming addicted.

    D. People whose parents have addiction problems are at greater risk of becoming addicts themselves.

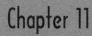

Practice Test

Completion: *Write the term that completes the statement in the space provided.*

1. Over-the-counter medications are sold to people without a _____ from a doctor or other licensed healthcare professional.

2. Aspirin, acetaminophen, and ibuprofen are examples of _____, or pain relievers.

3. Drowsiness, dizziness, weakness, nausea, confusion, and internal bleeding are examples of _____ that can result from the use of some medications.

4. _____ is any use of medication that does not follow the medication's instructions.

5. _____ involves the intentional use of medications for purposes other than those intended by the prescribing doctor.

True/False: *Indicate whether each statement below is true or false by circling either T or F.*

T   F   6. Opioids are typically prescribed to relieve itching.

T   F   7. Depressants are used to relieve anxiety and increase a person's ability to relax and stay calm.

T   F   8. Stimulants increase the level of dopamine in the brain, producing a feeling of euphoria.

T   F   9. Over-the-counter medications intended for adults can always be given to infants and children.

T   F   10. Stimulants are commonly prescribed for people with ADHD.

Multiple Choice: *Write the letter that corresponds to the correct answer in the blank space.*

_____ 11. The Food and Drug Administration (FDA) ensures that medications are _____, effective, and secure from tampering.
   A. safe
   B. approved for in-flight transit
   C. delivered to pharmacies in a timely manner
   D. kept in a cool, dark location until they are used

_____ 12. A chemical called _____ is the active ingredient in marijuana.
   A. opium
   B. lysergic acid diethylamide
   C. delta-9-tetrahydrocannabinol (THC)
   D. Cannabis

_____ 13. _____ are drugs that cause people to see, hear, or feel things that are not real.
   A. Muscle relaxants
   B. Anabolic steroids
   C. Bath salts
   D. Hallucinogens

(Continued)

_____ 14. Some people illegally use _____ to gain strength and increase their muscle size.
   A. anabolic steroids
   B. inhalants
   C. club drugs
   D. opioids

_____ 15. _____ is a condition that occurs when the supply of oxygen needed by the body is depleted.
   A. Euphoria
   B. Hypoxia
   C. Paranoia
   D. Memory loss

Matching: *Match each key term to its definition by writing the letter of the term in the space provided.*

_____ 16. form of addiction in which a person's body requires a drug to function normally

_____ 17. use of drugs by an individual to treat problems and symptoms not diagnosed by a medical doctor

_____ 18. unpleasant side effects that people may experience when they try to stop taking a drug

_____ 19. the act of using drugs excessively or without medical reason

_____ 20. houses or communities that provide alcohol- and drug-free living environments for people who are trying to abstain from substance use

_____ 21. the ingestion of more of a drug than the body can successfully process, or break down

_____ 22. a state in which increasingly larger amounts of a drug are required to achieve the same good feelings

_____ 23. process used in treatment programs to clear all drugs from a person's body

_____ 24. the emotional distress that arises when people with a drug addiction feel that they need a drug to function normally

A. drug abuse

B. drug overdose

C. physical addiction

D. psychological addiction

E. withdrawal

F. self-medication

G. detoxification

H. tolerance

I. sober living community

Short Answer: *On a separate sheet of paper, answer the following questions using what you have learned in this chapter.*

25. Drug abuse has negative consequences, both for individuals struggling with addiction and for addicts' families, friends, and coworkers. Describe the broader impact that drug abuse and addiction have on society.

26. Outline the steps you would take if you discovered that a close friend was addicted to drugs. Start by considering the first thing you would do.

Lesson 12.1

Key Concepts Review

Multiple Choice: *Write the letter that corresponds to the correct answer in the blank space.*

_____ 1. Which of the following is *not* a communicable disease?
A. pneumonia
B. influenza
C. cancer
D. strep throat

_____ 2. _____ is the scientific concept that specific microorganisms cause specific diseases.
A. Germ theory
B. Pathology postulate
C. Infection supposition
D. Disease principle

_____ 3. Which type of disease is caused by microorganisms living in or on humans, animals, or plants?
A. noncommunicable disease
B. infectious disease
C. macroorganism disease
D. food poisoning

_____ 4. What is another term for *communicable disease*?
A. fungal disease
B. conversable disease
C. infectious disease
D. parasitic pandemic

_____ 5. _____ are evidence of disease that can be outwardly observed or measured.
A. Signs
B. Symptoms
C. Indicators
D. Alterations

_____ 6. Which type of bacteria makes toxins that disrupt the ability of intestines to absorb water?
A. chicken pox
B. barbiturates
C. Salmonella
D. pneumonia

_____ 7. Which of the following are examples of microorganisms?
A. bacteria
B. viruses
C. fungi
D. all of the above

_____ 8. What is the technical term for the time period between the entrance of a pathogen into the body and the first appearance of signs and symptoms?
A. incubation period
B. infestation period
C. infiltration period
D. invasion period

_____ 9. During which stage of an illness or a disease do characteristic signs and symptoms arise?
A. pathogenic stage
B. incubation stage
C. clinical stage
D. manifestation stage

_____ 10. During this stage of illness, the immune system has destroyed the invading pathogen, signs and symptoms of the illness fade, and a person is no longer contagious.
A. stage of resistance
B. convalescent stage
C. quiescent stage
D. acquiescent stage

Matching: *Match each microorganism to its characteristics by writing the letter of the microorganism in the blank space.*

_____ 11. Examples of this type of microorganism include mushrooms, molds, and yeast.

_____ 12. Most of these microorganisms are helpful to the human body; few of them cause disease.

_____ 13. This category of microorganisms consists of protozoa and worms.

_____ 14. These microorganisms depend entirely on other cells for reproduction and growth.

A. bacteria

B. viruses

C. fungi

D. parasites

Signs and Symptoms

The terms signs *and* symptoms *are often confused.* Signs *are objective evidence of illness or disease that can be outwardly observed or measured. Examples of signs are fever, abnormal pulse, changes in skin color, or an altered breathing rate. By contrast,* symptoms *are subjective evidence of illness or disease sensed by the sick person. Examples of symptoms are pain, shortness of breath, itching, or headache.*

For each medical scenario presented below, differentiate between the signs and symptoms for each patient. If a patient does not exhibit either signs or symptoms, write "N/A" in the appropriate column.

Scenario	Signs	Symptoms
1. Michael has a headache, fever (temperature of 101° F), chills, and a sore throat.		
2. LaShara has nasal and sinus congestion, and she has been sneezing and coughing.		
3. Following a vigorous game of basketball, Alan feels cold, clammy, and nauseous, and his skin appears pale.		
4. Mary recently got her ears pierced. One of her ears has begun to bleed. In addition, the ear looks red and inflamed, and Mary is experiencing mild pain.		
5. Harrison has been experiencing extreme thirst and frequent urination. Once mildly obese, he has lost 30 pounds in two months without trying to lose weight.		
6. As Dorothy was walking her dog, her dog spotted a squirrel and lunged in its direction. Dorothy felt a "popping" sound in her shoulder, followed by a sharp pain and an inability to raise her arm.		

Lesson 12.1

Autobiography of a Pathogen

You are a well-known author of books for children between the ages of 8 and 11. Last night, your literary agent called to inform you that your publisher, Hill Academy Press, has proposed that you write an entertaining and informative children's story about the journey of a pathogen through the human body. The subject of your story may be a bacterium, virus, fungus, or parasite; and the tale should be autobiographical—that is, told from the pathogen's point of view. Your literary agent explains that Hill Academy Press will hire a qualified artist to pair whimsical drawings with your creative prose. To help you get started, your agent submits the following questions to you. Answer each of her questions in the space below.

1. Who is the main character of your story: a bacterium, virus, fungus, or parasite? What is his or her name?

   _____

2. What is the plot of your story? For example, is your bacterium a "good guy or girl"? Will she or he be engaged in battle against harmful bacteria to protect the immune system of your human host? Will your pathogen be a villain?

   _____
   _____
   _____
   _____
   _____
   _____

3. What is the theme, or central idea, of your story? Will it be, for example, perseverance in overcoming obstacles? Is your character on a "personal" mission to accomplish a goal? If so, what is that mission? Why is the mission important to your character?

   _____
   _____
   _____
   _____
   _____
   _____

4. How will your story end?

   _____
   _____
   _____
   _____
   _____
   _____

After you have answered your agent's questions, write the personal story of your pathogen in one or two pages using separate sheets of paper. (You may write a longer piece if you wish.)

Name _____ Date _____

Finding Reliable Health Information

For this activity, you will find three sources of reliable information for each of the three topics listed below. You may use the sources of information given in Figure 1.6, "Health and Safety Information," or you may research your own sources. For each source, write the name of the organization and the title of the article or web page. If the source does not appear in Figure 1.6, list its website address as well. Do not use a source more than once.

Topic: *MRSA (methicillin-resistant Staphylococcus aureus)*

1. A. Website #1 (name of organization) _____

   B. Title of article or web page _____

2. A. Website #2 (name of organization) _____

   B. Title of article or web page _____

3. A. Website #3 (name of organization) _____

   B. Title of article or web page _____

Topic: *Meningitis*

1. A. Website #1 (name of organization) _____

   B. Title of article or web page _____

2. A. Website #2 (name of organization) _____

   B. Title of article or web page _____

3. A. Website #3 (name of organization) _____

   B. Title of article or web page _____

Topic: *Mononucleosis*

1. A. Website #1 (name of organization) _____

   B. Title of article or web page _____

2. A. Website #2 (name of organization) _____

   B. Title of article or web page _____

3. A. Website #3 (name of organization) _____

   B. Title of article or web page _____

After compiling the above information about your sources, answer the following questions:

1. Of the three sources you chose for each topic, which sources were most reliable? How do you know?

_____

_____

2. Which sources provided the most interesting information? Write three facts you learned about each topic.

_____

_____

Lesson 12.3

Key Term Scramble

Unscramble each key term in the first column. In the second column, write the definition of the unscrambled key term.

Term	Definition
y o d i n t a b	
c v c a n i e	
a i c l i	
f r e e v	
c u u m s	
f l i n t a m i n a m o	
c h o g y a p e t	

Chapter 12

Scientific and Medical Terms

Many scientific and medical terms in the English language consist of word parts from Latin and/or Greek. Each word listed below appears in one or more lessons in chapter 12. Beside each term, you will see its Greek or Latin root word(s), plus other word parts that help make up the term. A meaning has been provided for each word part.

Read each term and the meanings of its word parts. Then, based on these word parts, write the definition of each term. (The first one has been done for you.) When you are finished, look up the terms in a dictionary or in your textbook's glossary, and compare those definitions with the ones that you wrote.

Term	Word Parts	Meanings	Definition
1. antibiotic	anti- bi/o -tic	against life pertaining to	pertaining to (being) against life *(An antibiotic is a substance that fights "against life"—specifically, against bacterial microorganisms.)*
2. endemic	en- dem/o -ic	within people pertaining to	
3. epidemic	epi- dem/o -ic	above; upon people pertaining to	
4. immunity	immun/o -ity	safe; protection quality, state, or degree	
5. microorganism	micro- organ/o -ism	small organ condition	

Name _____

Term	Word Parts	Meanings	Definition
6. pandemic	pan- dem/o -ic	all people pertaining to	
7. parasite	para- sit/o	near; beside; alongside food	
8. pathogen	path/o -gen	disease substance that produces	
9. phagocyte	phag/o -cyte	eat; swallow; engulf cell	
10. pneumonia	pneumon/o -ia	lung state; condition	
11. protozoa	prot/o zo/o -a	first animal life plural suffix	
12. zoonosis	zo/o -(n)osis	animal life abnormal condition	

Name ______________________________ Date ______________

Chapter 12

Reading Practice

Reread the following passage from the textbook. Then answer the questions on the next page.

Treatment for Infectious Diseases

Until the 1940s, there were no antibiotics to treat bacterial infections. Today, medical science has developed effective treatments that have decreased suffering and death caused by infectious disease. In some cases, an infection overwhelms the body's defenses. When that happens, you can take certain medications that will kill the infection-causing pathogens. Such medications also shorten the disease's duration, reducing the chance that a disease will cause lasting damage.

Treating Bacterial Infections

Naturally made by fungi and helpful bacteria, ***antibiotics*** are substances that target and kill pathogenic bacteria. Antibiotics are effective against many kinds of pathogenic bacteria, but it is important to know that they are ineffective against viruses, fungi, and parasites.

Most antibiotics, such as penicillin, erythromycin, and amoxicillin, are prescription medications. A doctor must order these for a patient to buy from a pharmacist. These antibiotics are typically taken as pills or capsules. For some serious infections, antibiotics might be injected or infused directly into veins. These are called *intravenous* or *IV antibiotics.*

A few antibiotics are available "over-the-counter"—they can be purchased at drugstores without a doctor's prescription. Examples include creams with bacitracin or neomycin for treating minor cuts and scrapes.

Unfortunately, several strains of bacteria have developed ***antibiotic resistance***. An antibiotic resistant bacterium cannot be killed by antibiotics. These strains of bacteria are extremely difficult, if not impossible, to treat because the antibiotics once used are no longer effective. For example, ***MRSA (methicillin-resistant Staphylococcus aureus)*** is a strain of ordinary S. aureus that cannot be controlled with many antibiotics.

Antibiotic resistance is both a personal and public health problem. It can be avoided by taking the following precautions:

- Use antibiotics only when prescribed.
- Do not share antibiotics.
- Do not take antibiotics for viral infections.
- Take the entire dose for the length of time prescribed by your doctor.

Treating Viral Infections

There are few treatments for viral infections. Most medications target the symptoms and do not attack the virus. In many cases, medicines treat the signs and symptoms of disease, with the goal of making you more comfortable. That is the purpose of medicines like acetaminophen, which reduces fever, aches, and pains associated with influenza. Cough medicines, decongestants, anti-inflammatories, and antihistamines treat various symptoms, but provide no cures.

For infections such as genital herpes, hepatitis, and severe influenza, drugs can reduce the severity of the infection, but do not cure these viral infections. In these cases, the drugs keep the virus under control while the body fights back. Rest, good nutrition, and fluids strengthen the body and help it fight the virus.

There are also several drugs that control and cure infections caused by worms and protozoan parasites.

Name_____ Date _____

_____ 1. In what decade did antibiotics become available to treat bacterial infections?
   A. 1940s
   B. 1950s
   C. 1960s
   D. 1970s

_____ 2. Antibiotics, substances that target and kill pathogenic bacteria, are naturally made by which of the following microorganisms?
   A. steroids
   B. parasites
   C. fungi and helpful bacteria
   D. none of the above

_____ 3 . Which of the following is an accurate description of *antibiotic resistance*?
   A. prescription of an antibiotic for any illness other than a bacterial infection
   B. the ability of a bacterium to "fight back" against an antibiotic
   C. reduced effectiveness of an intravenous antibiotic
   D. resistance of a bacterium to bacitracin or neomycin

_____ 4. Antibiotic resistance can be avoided by taking which of the following precautions?
   A. using antibiotics only when prescribed
   B. taking the entire dose of an antibiotic for the length of time prescribed by a doctor
   C. not taking antibiotics for viral infections
   D. all of the above

_____ 5. _____ are antibiotics that are injected or infused directly into the veins.
   A. Over-the-counter antibiotics
   B. Liquid antibiotics
   C. Intravenous antibiotics
   D. none of the above

_____ 6. Which of the following statements is true about medications used to treat viral infections?
   A. Most medications target the virus and do not relieve the symptoms.
   B. Most medications target the symptoms and do not attack the virus.
   C. Most medications worsen the symptoms while attacking the virus.
   D. Most medications alleviate the symptoms as they target the virus.

_____ 7. _____ can be treated with medication to reduce its severity but cannot be cured.
   A. Influenza virus
   B. Hepatitis virus
   C. Genital herpes virus
   D. all of the above

Chapter 12

Practice Test

Completion: *Write the term that completes the statement in the space provided.*

1. Infectious diseases are caused by _____ living in or on humans, animals, or plants.

2. Microorganisms that cause disease are known as _____.

3. Infectious diseases, also called _____, are caused by pathogens that can be transmitted from one living thing to another.

4. Diseases not caused by pathogens are called _____ diseases.

5. _____ are evidence of disease that can be outwardly observed or measured.

6. _____ are evidence of disease sensed by a sick person; they are subjective and cannot be easily seen or measured by other people.

True/False: *Indicate whether each statement below is true or false by circling either T or F.*

T   F   7. Evidence of a disease that is observable and measurable is called *subjective* evidence.

T   F   8. Evidence of a disease that is not easily observed and measured is called *objective* evidence.

T   F   9. The *incubation period* is the time between a pathogen's entrance into the body and the first appearance of symptoms.

T   F   10. During the *clinical stage*, a pathogen produces toxins and the immune response reaches its height, causing familiar signs of illness.

T   F   11. In the *convalescent stage*, signs and symptoms of an illness gradually worsen.

T   F   12. Most bacteria are not harmful to the body.

T   F   13. Bacteria, viruses, fungi, and phagocytes are examples of pathogens.

T   F   14. Bacterial cells make up 90% of cells in the human body.

T   F   15. *Escherichia coli* (*E. coli*) is a bacterium that resides in animal and human intestines and causes food poisoning.

Multiple Choice: *Write the letter that corresponds to the correct answer in the blank space.*

_____ 16. Which of the following is true about viruses?

    A. Viruses do not grow or reproduce independently.

    B. Viruses have no metabolism.

    C. Viruses do not use energy in the way that other cells do.

    D. all of the above

_____ 17. Which of the following is the plural form of *fungus*?

    A. funguses

    B. fungi

    C. fungii

    D. fungae

_____ 18. Mycosis, which usually attacks damaged tissues or people weakened by other infections, is described as a(n) _____.

    A. intestinal infection

    B. parasitic infection

    C. opportunistic infection

    D. infiltrative infection

_____ 19. Which of the following is *not* an example of a fungus?
- A. *Streptococcus pyogenes*
- B. *Cryptococcus neoformans*
- C. *Penicillium notatum*
- D. *Pneumocystis jirovecii*

_____ 20. Parasitic worms are _____ organisms with specialized tissues and organs.
- A. single-celled
- B. quadricellular
- C. pentacellular
- D. multicellular

Matching: *Match each key term to its definition by writing the letter of the term in the space provided.*

_____ 21. a strain of *S. aureus* that is highly resistant to antibiotic control

_____ 22. a substance that targets and destroys pathogenic bacteria

_____ 23. an infectious disease that is transmitted from animals to humans

_____ 24. an infection that impacts an enormous number of people as it spreads from one country to much of the world

_____ 25. an infection that occurs in unexpectedly large numbers over a particular area

_____ 26. simple actions taken to prevent the spread of communicable diseases

_____ 27. a process by which a person's immune system becomes active, rendering the body immune from a disease

_____ 28. the ability of some strains of bacteria to "fight back" against antibiotics

_____ 29. an organism that transmits disease from one living thing to another; examples include flies, mosquitoes, ticks, and fleas

_____ 30. a dead pathogen, or a nontoxic component of a pathogen, that is injected into the body, where it stimulates production of white blood cells, proteins, and chemicals to provide immunity against disease

_____ 31. an infection that naturally occurs at low levels in a particular area

_____ 32. a food sanitation practice in which pathogens are destroyed by heating foods and beverages to certain temperatures and then quickly cooling them

_____ 33. a simple practice that is universally acknowledged to be the most important method of preventing many infectious diseases

- A. antibiotic
- B. antibiotic resistance
- C. endemic
- D. epidemic
- E. hand washing
- F. MRSA (methicillin-resistant *Staphylococcus aureus*)
- G. pandemic
- H. pasteurization
- I. respiratory etiquette
- J. vaccine
- K. immunization
- L. vector
- M. zoonosis

Short Answer: *On a separate sheet of paper, answer the following questions using what you have learned in this chapter.*

34. Explain why the body's integumentary system, the *skin*, is the "first line of defense" against infection. Describe ways in which the skin protects the body from infectious invaders.

35. Briefly define the term *vaccine* and give at least three examples of vaccines.

36. Summarize the difference between the *direct transmission* and *indirect transmission* of an infectious disease. Give two examples of each transmission method.

Lesson 13.1

STI Transmission

The transmission of STIs can be an issue of great concern for teens and adults who want to maintain their health. As their name suggests, sexually transmitted infections (STIs) are most often transmitted during sexual activity. There are protective methods that can be used to prevent the transmission of STIs, but these methods are not always effective. In each of the following scenarios, identify whether an STI could have been transmitted or not.

1. Brandy and Jim have been friends for years and have just begun dating. The night after Brandy and Jim kiss for the first time, Brandy texts her best friend to tell her the exciting news. Brandy's best friend wants to be excited for her, but she also has some bad news. She heard that Jim has a sexually transmitted infection known as *genital herpes*, which can sometimes manifest as sores on the mouth. Could an STI have been transmitted? Why or why not?

   _____

   _____

   _____

   _____

   _____

2. Twenty-eight-year-old Travis and twenty-five-year-old Tina have been engaged for a few years. They've discussed the topic of sexual activity and eventually decide that they are both ready. During their discussions, Travis reveals that he has been sexually active in the past and that a recent test showed he has an STI known as *syphilis*. When they engage in sexual intercourse, Travis and Tina use a latex condom. Could an STI be transmitted? Why or why not?

   _____

   _____

   _____

   _____

   _____

3. Beth and Jen are hanging out at their friend David's house. While there, Beth uses the bathroom. After they leave David's house, Jen tells Beth that David has an STI. Beth is worried because she used the same toilet seat that David has used in the past. Could an STI have been transmitted? Why or why not?

   _____

   _____

   _____

   _____

   _____

Lesson 13.1

Practicing Abstinence

Sexual abstinence is the decision to refrain from sexual activity. There are many reasons why people choose to practice abstinence. It may be part of a person's values or religious beliefs; or a person may choose abstinence because he or she is not ready to engage in sexual activity. What's more, abstinence is the only method that is 100% effective at preventing STIs. Whatever the reason, a person's choice to practice abstinence should always be respected. Those who choose abstinence often face challenges to their choices, from friends, society, or the media. In many cases, people will need to use refusal skills to maintain their commitments to abstinence. Read the following scenarios in which a person's choice to practice abstinence is being challenged. In each situation, provide an example of a strong response that would convey how serious each person is about his or her choice to abstain from sexual activity.

1. Shondra and her boyfriend, Marcus, have been dating for two years. When the relationship first began, Shondra was clear about her choice to practice abstinence. Marcus seemed to agree with her at first, but then he began pressuring her to engage in sexual activity. He tells Shondra that she should be ready by now since they have been dating for several years. How should Shondra respond?

   _____

   _____

   _____

2. Jared and Marina have been dating all throughout high school. Although Jared knows that his relationship with Marina is solid and that they may get married while in college, he has chosen to remain abstinent until marriage. Marina and Jared have discussed this before, and Marina has always seemed to agree with Jared. Graduation is approaching, however, and many of Marina's friends are talking about having sex with their dates on prom night. Marina mentions this idea to Jared. What should he say?

   _____

   _____

   _____

3. Bonnie and Clive have only been on four dates. Bonnie is committed to abstinence, but she has not yet had a discussion about it with Clive. One evening, when they're coming home from the movie theater, Clive mentions that his parents are away for the weekend. He invites Bonnie over to his house to stay the night and implies that he would like to engage in sexual activity. Bonnie wants to hang out with Clive, but she doesn't want to put herself in a risky situation. What should Bonnie say?

   _____

   _____

   _____

4. Hannah and Toby have been dating all through high school. All of Hannah's friends are dating as well, and they often talk about their dates together. One day, Hannah's friends start discussing how they've already had sex with their boyfriends. Hannah's friends ask why Hannah and Toby haven't. Hannah and Toby have already talked about this and have both decided to remain abstinent. How could Hannah explain this to her friends?

   _____

   _____

   _____

Lesson 13.1

Finding Reliable Health Information

For this activity, you will find three sources of reliable information for each of the three topics listed below. You may use the sources of information given in Figure 1.6, "Health and Safety Information," or you may research your own sources. For each source, write the name of the organization and the title of the article or web page. If the source does not appear in Figure 1.6, list its website address as well. Do not use a source more than once.

Topic: *Health problems associated with STIs*

1. A. Website #1 (name of organization) _____

   B. Title of article or web page _____

2. A. Website #2 (name of organization) _____

   B. Title of article or web page _____

3. A. Website #3 (name of organization) _____

   B. Title of article or web page _____

Topic: *STI treatments*

1. A. Website #1 (name of organization) _____

   B. Title of article or web page _____

2. A. Website #2 (name of organization) _____

   B. Title of article or web page _____

3. A. Website #3 (name of organization) _____

   B. Title of article or web page _____

Topic: *STI prevention*

1. A. Website #1 (name of organization) _____

   B. Title of article or web page _____

2. A. Website #2 (name of organization) _____

   B. Title of article or web page _____

3. A. Website #3 (name of organization) _____

   B. Title of article or web page _____

After compiling the above information about your sources, answer the following questions:

1. Of the three sources you chose for each topic, which sources were most reliable? How do you know?

   _____

   _____

2. Which sources provided the most interesting information? Write three facts you learned about each topic.

   _____

   _____

Lesson 13.2

STI Quiz

Multiple Choice: *Write the letter that corresponds to the correct answer in the blank space.*

_____ 1. There are about _____ new cases of sexually transmitted infections reported in the United States each year.

    A. 14,100,000   C. 20,000,000

    B. 1,090,000   D. 776,000

_____ 2. _____ is a bacterial STI that can be fatal if not treated.

    A. Trachoma   C. Chlamydia

    B. Syphilis   D. Pelvic inflammatory disease

_____ 3. More than 1,400,000 cases of _____, known as the *silent disease*, are reported per year in the United States.

    A. syphilis   C. gonorrhea

    B. chlamydia   D. HPV

_____ 4. _____ is a curable STI that may cause burning or itching, but is usually asymptomatic.

    A. Trichomoniasis   C. Herpes

    B. Syphilis   D. Gonorrhea

_____ 5. Outbreaks of sores sometimes accompanied by a fever are caused by _____.

    A. syphilis   C. pelvic inflammatory disease

    B. gonorrhea   D. genital herpes

_____ 6. Women with _____ may experience mild burning or itching that seems like a vaginal yeast infection.

    A. pelvic inflammatory disease   C. gonorrhea

    B. syphilis   D. genital warts

_____ 7. _____ is the most commonly contracted STI.

    A. Human papillomavirus   C. Syphilis

    B. Herpes simplex virus   D. Trichomoniasis

_____ 8. If a woman with pelvic inflammatory disease becomes pregnant, she may develop a(n) _____ pregnancy.

    A. undiagnosed   C. trichomoniasis

    B. ectopic   D. viral

_____ 9. Which of the following STIs is *not* treated with antibiotics?

    A. syphilis   C. gonorrhea

    B. chlamydia   D. genital warts

_____ 10. Human papillomavirus can cause _____ cancer and oropharyngeal cancer.

    A. cervical   C. prostate

    B. ovarian   D. pelvic

Lesson 13.2

STI Test Results

Each sexually transmitted infection has its own set of symptoms and treatments. Knowing the specific symptoms a patient has can help a doctor or nurse identify which STI the patient has contracted. Imagine that you are a doctor who is diagnosing a patient with an STI. Read each of the following descriptions of a patient's symptoms. Then diagnose each person with an STI and explain what type of treatment is best suited for that specific STI.

1. Bianca has a copper-colored rash on the palms of her hands and the soles of her feet. When asked, she reveals that she noticed a painless sore on her tongue three weeks ago. In addition to her rash, Bianca feels fatigued and has a mild fever. After an examination, you note that Bianca's lymph nodes are swollen.

   A. Which STI does Bianca have?

   _____

   B. What treatments are available?

   _____

   _____

2. Gabby has noticed warts on her genitals and she tells you that she has been having unprotected sex with her boyfriend. She is worried that she has contracted an STI like herpes. You are concerned about the genital warts, so you perform a Pap smear.

   A. Which STI does Gabby have?

   _____

   B. What treatments are available?

   _____

   _____

3. Greg has noticed sores on his genitals. In the past, he has only had these types of sores on his mouth. He always thought they were just cold sores, but now he is concerned. Greg tells you that he had a mild fever the last time he noticed one of these cold sores on his lip.

   A. Which STI does Greg have?

   _____

   B. What treatments are available?

   _____

   _____

4. Cathy has started experiencing nausea, abdominal pain, fever, and abnormal bleeding during her menstrual period. She recently read about HPV infection and thinks she may have contracted that when she had unprotected sex last summer. Until now, she has not experienced any symptoms.

   A. Which STI does Cathy have?

   _____

   B. What treatments are available?

   _____

   _____

Lesson 13.3

HIV Transmission

HIV transmission is a source of concern for many people who want to protect their health. Understanding which bodily fluids can transmit HIV is important for knowing whether you are at risk for contracting the virus. Read the following scenarios and determine whether the person should be worried about HIV transmission. Explain your answer.

1. Heather's uncle has HIV/AIDS. After visiting, Heather's uncle kisses her good-bye on the cheek. Should Heather and her uncle be concerned about HIV transmission? Explain.

   _____

   _____

   _____

   _____

2. Bill knows that Harry, a person who works out at his gym, has HIV/AIDS. One day Bill uses exercise equipment that Harry has just used, and he notices the equipment is covered with Harry's sweat. Should Bill and Harry be concerned about HIV transmission? Explain.

   _____

   _____

   _____

   _____

3. Diane has a daughter named Isabelle. After Isabelle was born, Diane contracted HIV/AIDS. Diane thinks that breast-feeding is important, so she continues to breast-feed Isabelle after her diagnosis. Should Diane be concerned about HIV transmission? Explain.

   _____

   _____

   _____

   _____

4. Valerie and Hank have been friends for many years, and Valerie knows that Hank has HIV/AIDS. After going on a run together, Hank and Valerie share a water bottle to rehydrate themselves. Should Valerie and Hank be concerned about HIV transmission? Explain.

   _____

   _____

   _____

   _____

5. John has HIV/AIDS. Jill and John have sexual intercourse and do not use a condom or other protective method. Should Jill and John be concerned about HIV transmission? Explain.

   _____

   _____

   _____

   _____

Lesson 13.3

HIV/AIDS Quiz

Multiple Choice: *Write the letter that corresponds to the correct answer in the blank space.*

_____ 1. A person is said to be _____ if a laboratory test detects the presence of HIV antibodies in the person's blood.
   A. HIV-infected
   B. HIV-positive
   C. HIV-viral
   D. HIV-negative

_____ 2. Early symptoms of HIV/AIDS resemble _____ with fatigue and swollen, painful lymph nodes.
   A. the flu
   B. chlamydia
   C. gonorrhea
   D. hypothermia

_____ 3. _____ is a virus that infects and kills cells, thus weakening the body's immune system.
   A. AIDS
   B. Trichomoniasis
   C. HIV
   D. Gonorrhea

_____ 4. _____ is an often fatal disease in which the body's immune system can no longer fight off infections and diseases.
   A. AIDS
   B. Trichomoniasis
   C. HIV
   D. Gonorrhea

_____ 5. People with AIDS are vulnerable to many infections, including _____.
   A. tuberculosis
   B. thrush
   C. Kaposi's sarcoma
   D. all of the above

_____ 6. HIV-positive people whose infections progress to AIDS slowly are known as _____.
   A. T-helpers
   B. non-transmitters
   C. long-term non-progressors
   D. untested HIV patients

_____ 7. Having other _____ increases one's risk for becoming infected with HIV.
   A. STIs
   B. health problems
   C. infections
   D. illnesses

_____ 8. _____ infections take advantage of a weakened body and are often the cause of death in HIV/AIDS patients.
   A. Sexually transmitted
   B. Blood
   C. Undiagnosed
   D. Opportunistic

_____ 9. Treatment for HIV/AIDS is known as _____ therapy, or a *cocktail of drugs*.
   A. radiation
   B. anti-retroviral
   C. viral
   D. chemical

_____ 10. HIV tests and results are kept _____ if requested.
   A. publicly available
   B. rapid
   C. inexpensive
   D. confidential

Name _____ Date _____

Sexual Health Careers

In the *Spotlight on Health and Wellness Careers* feature in this chapter, several careers that relate to sexual health are discussed. When choosing a healthcare career, you should be mindful of your personal interests, strengths, and weaknesses. These will help you decide which career would best suit you. Study the chart below, which is organized according to interest or personal quality, and then answer the questions on the next page. Keep in mind your own interests, strengths, and weaknesses when reviewing the chart.

Interest/Quality	Career	Duties	Education and Training	Resources
Enjoys working with the public	Medical Laboratory Technologist	Collects samples from patients	Bachelor's degree, certification, or licensure	American Society for Clinical Laboratory Science
	Community Health Worker	Conducts community outreach programs	Associate's degree and/or certification	American Public Health Association
Enjoys working with data or paperwork	Health Information Technician	Organizes, maintains, and records patient health data	Associate's degree and/or certification	American Health Information Management Association
	Medical Laboratory Technologist	Analyzes patients' blood and tissue specimens	Bachelor's degree, certification, or licensure	American Society for Clinical Laboratory Science
	Microbiologist	Studies microorganisms and records data	Bachelor's degree and/or master's degree or Ph.D.	American Society for Microbiology
Is interested in science	Microbiologist	Studies microorganisms, such as those that cause STIs	Bachelor's degree and/or master's degree or Ph.D.	American Society for Microbiology
	Medical Laboratory Technologist	Analyzes blood and tissue samples	Bachelor's degree, certification, or licensure	American Society for Clinical Laboratory Science
Enjoys working in a fast-paced environment	Medical Laboratory Technologist	Collects samples, performs tests, and analyzes results in a timely manner	Bachelor's degree, certification, or licensure	American Society for Clinical Laboratory Science
Is able to meet deadlines	Microbiologist	Presents data and findings in a timely manner	Bachelor's degree and/or master's degree or Ph.D.	American Society for Microbiology
Enjoys working independently	Health Information Technician	Works with patient data rather than with patients	Associate's degree and/or certification	American Health Information Management Association
	Microbiologist	Spends time analyzing data in the lab	Bachelor's degree and/or master's degree or Ph.D.	American Society for Microbiology
Has good communication skills	Health Information Technician	Reports cases of STIs per hospital guidelines	Associate's degree and/or certification	American Health Information Management Association
	Community Health Worker	Educates the public about health concerns	Associate's degree and/or certification	American Public Health Association

(Continued)

1. Which of these careers lines up best with your interests or personality?

   _____
   _____
   _____
   _____

2. Choose one career to research further. For that career, visit the resource listed in the chart and compose a "day in the life" for someone with that career. Does this type of workday sound interesting to you?

   _____
   _____
   _____
   _____
   _____
   _____
   _____

3. According to the chart, which level of education is necessary for your chosen career? Research community colleges and universities in your area and plot out an educational plan to follow if you want this career.

   _____
   _____
   _____
   _____

4. Visit the *Occupational Outlook Handbook* online to research the job outlook for this particular career. Record your findings here.

   _____
   _____
   _____
   _____
   _____
   _____

5. According to the *Occupational Outlook Handbook*, what is a typical salary for someone in this career?

   _____
   _____
   _____
   _____

Chapter 13

Reading Practice

Reread the following passage from the textbook. Then answer the questions that follow.

STIs Cause Serious Health Problems

STIs are caused by infectious microorganisms, which cause many health problems. Bacteria produce toxins that damage organs, and most infectious microorganisms trigger inflammation. *Inflammation* is the body's reaction to infection. When inflammation occurs, a body part may become red, warm, swollen, or painful. Inflammation often occurs in body parts affected by an STI.

People with STIs are often ***asymptomatic***, which means they exhibit few or no symptoms of disease. Asymptomatic people do have the disease, however, and they do carry the bacteria or viruses. This means they can also transmit the disease to others primarily through sexual acts. Additionally, having no symptoms does not mean that health problems are not occurring in an infected person.

While some STIs cause little or no discomfort, these diseases can still damage the reproductive organs and cause *infertility*, the inability to conceive and have children. For example, two of the STIs you will read about in the next lesson can scar the *fallopian tubes*, which normally deliver fertilized eggs to the uterus. In fact, people can develop infertility or other permanent health problems even if they have been cured of an STI.

_____ 1. What is the main idea of this passage?
   A. If a disease is asymptomatic, that means few or no symptoms can be detected.
   B. STIs can cause many health problems.
   C. STIs can cause damage to reproductive organs.
   D. Inflammation is the body's reaction to infection.

_____ 2. Which of the following terms describes the inability to conceive and have children?
   A. asymptomatic
   B. inflammation
   C. cured
   D. infertility

_____ 3. What is the term for reproductive organs that deliver fertilized eggs to the uterus?
   A. infertility
   B. fallopian tubes
   C. passageway
   D. toxins

_____ 4. Which of the following is a common side effect of sexually transmitted infections?
   A. inflammation
   B. asymptomatic
   C. transmission
   D. abstinence

Chapter 13

Practice Test

Completion: *Write the term that completes the statement in the space provided.*

1. Even asymptomatic STIs can damage the reproductive organs and cause
   _____.

2. A _____ can provide a barrier to microorganisms that cause STIs.

3. _____ is also known as the *great imitator*.

4. The _____ is normally used to screen for cervical cancer, which is caused by HPV.

5. Blood tests show that HIV specifically destroys _____ cells.

True/False: *Indicate whether each statement below is true or false by circling either T or F.*

T   F   6. Engaging in sexual activity one time with just one infected partner is all it takes to contract an STI.

T   F   7. Chlamydia does *not* affect a woman's reproductive health.

T   F   8. An HIV-positive person who has other STIs more easily transmits those STIs to sexual partners.

T   F   9. Late-stage syphilis does *not* include obvious external signs.

T   F   10. There are no laws to protect people with HIV/AIDS from discrimination.

Multiple Choice: *Write the letter that corresponds to the correct answer in the blank space.*

_____ 11. Sexual _____ is the only method that is 100% effective in preventing STIs.
  A. prevention   C. treatment
  B. abstinence   D. infection

_____ 12. _____ do nothing to prevent sexually transmitted infections.
  A. Condoms   C. Birth control pills
  B. Refusal skills   D. Abstinence skills

_____ 13. Which of the following STIs has about 55,000 cases reported each year in the US?
  A. syphilis   C. chlamydia
  B. HPV   D. trichomoniasis

_____ 14. Which of the following is *not* a stage of syphilis?
  A. secondary syphilis   C. congenital syphilis
  B. late-stage syphilis   D. primary syphilis

_____ 15. Which of the following is *not* a possible result of HPV?
  A. cervical cancer   C. oropharyngeal cancer
  B. genital warts   D. chancres

Name _____ Date _____

Matching: *Match each key term to its definition by writing the letter of the term in the space provided.*

_____ 16. an infection of the fallopian tubes and pelvic cavity

_____ 17. the quality of exhibiting no recognizable signs or symptoms of disease

_____ 18. a virus that infects and kills cells, thus weakening the body's immune system

_____ 19. a birth control device that provides a barrier to semen and microorganisms that cause STIs

_____ 20. an often fatal disease in which the body's immune system can no longer fight off infections and diseases

_____ 21. the most common STI, which infects and causes cells to grow abnormally

_____ 22. the decision and practice of refraining from sexual activity

A. abstinence

B. pelvic inflammatory disease

C. human papillomavirus (HPV)

D. acquired immunodeficiency syndrome (AIDS)

E. human immunodeficiency virus (HIV)

F. asymptomatic

G. latex condom

Analyzing Data: *The graph below illustrates the estimated number of new sexually transmitted infections in teens 15 to 24 years of age. Study the data in this graph and then answer the questions that follow.*

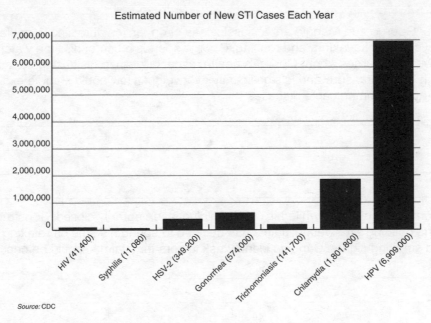

Estimated Number of New STI Cases Each Year

Source: CDC

23. Which STI had the most new cases? the least?

_____

24. In total, how many new cases of STIs were reported?

_____

25. What was the ratio of new HPV cases to new chlamydia cases?

_____

Short Answer: *On a separate sheet of paper, answer the following questions using what you have learned in this chapter.*

26. Why do you think it is important to keep HIV/AIDS test results confidential?

27. Do people die from HIV, AIDS, or complications associated with AIDS? Explain your answer.

Lesson 14.1

What Are the Risk Factors?

Each of the following scenarios describes a person who is at risk of developing a noncommunicable disease. Identify the specific risk factors for each individual. Then, categorize these risk factors as lifestyle-related, environmental, or hereditary.

1. At 65, Silvia has lived longer than either of her parents. Her father passed away when he was 60 from cancer, while her mother suffered a fatal stroke at age 64. A smoker for nearly 40 years, Silvia is very proud of herself for quitting last month. Although her doctors warn her that her high-fat diet may cause atherosclerosis, Silvia is sure she isn't at risk for any serious diseases. Can you identify any risk factors Silvia may be overlooking?

_____

_____

_____

_____

2. Married for 15 years, George and Maggie are a classic case of opposites attracting. Maggie eats healthfully and enjoys biking, kayaking, and running. George spends much of his time watching TV and has a sweet tooth. Maggie worries about George's health, especially since his last doctor appointment revealed he has high blood pressure and is significantly overweight. How could Maggie explain to George that he is at risk for a noncommunicable disease?

_____

_____

_____

_____

3. Jaime is enjoying some time off work while his office building is temporarily closed. Construction crews found asbestos in the building's insulation. Jaime has decided to spend his time off relaxing on his patio, reading a book, and smoking cigars. Can you identify risk factors that Jaime should be concerned about?

_____

_____

_____

_____

4. Ben recently celebrated his fiftieth birthday at a steakhouse with his family. For dinner, he had a porterhouse steak, asparagus, and a glass of red wine. Unfortunately, Ben's father, Jerry, was unable to attend the celebration because he was experiencing gout. Should Ben be concerned that he, too, may develop gout?

_____

_____

_____

_____

Lesson 14.2

Key Terms Review

Multiple Choice: *Write the letter that corresponds to the correct answer in the blank space.*

_____ 1. _____ are large, muscular blood vessels that transport blood from the heart to the capillaries.
    A. Arrhythmias   C. Arteries
    B. Veins   D. Valves

_____ 2. A hollow, wire mesh tube that is inserted into a blood vessel to restore blood flow is a(n) _____.
    A. artery   C. valve
    B. stent   D. angina

_____ 3. Which of the following are small, thin blood vessels that carry oxygen and nutrients from the arteries to the body's tissues?
    A. capillaries   C. aortas
    B. veins   D. arteries

_____ 4. The largest artery in the body is the _____.
    A. ventricle   C. coronary artery
    B. capillary   D. aorta

_____ 5. _____ are flaps of tissue that control blood flow in the heart.
    A. Ventricles   C. Valves
    B. Stents   D. Dilated ventricles

_____ 6. _____ are blood vessels that carry blood from the capillaries back to the heart.
    A. Veins   C. Coronary arteries
    B. Arteries   D. Arrhythmias

_____ 7. The force that blood exiting the heart exerts on the walls of the arteries is _____.
    A. angina   C. blood pressure
    B. hypertension   D. arrhythmia

_____ 8. Which of the following are blood vessels that deliver blood, oxygen, and nutrients to the heart?
    A. ventricles   C. veins
    B. capillaries   D. coronary arteries

_____ 9. _____ is also called high blood pressure.
    A. Hypertension   C. Stroke
    B. Atherosclerosis   D. Angina

Matching: *Write the letter of each disease in the blank next to its corresponding definition.*

_____ 10. an interruption of the blood flow to a section of the brain

_____ 11. a condition in which the heart weakens due to strain and becomes unable to successfully pump blood

_____ 12. a disease in which fatty substances collect on the walls of the arteries and restrict blood flow

_____ 13. a medical emergency in which the coronary arteries become blocked and restrict blood flow to the heart, causing the heart to beat irregularly and inefficiently

_____ 14. a disease of the blood vessels in which arteries harden and become unable to stretch, leading to high blood pressure and heart disease

A. congestive heart failure

B. heart attack

C. atherosclerosis

D. arteriosclerosis

E. stroke

Name _____ Date _____

Signs of a Heart Attack

Many different parts of the body can signal an upcoming heart attack. List the signs of a heart attack associated with each of the body parts on the figure below.

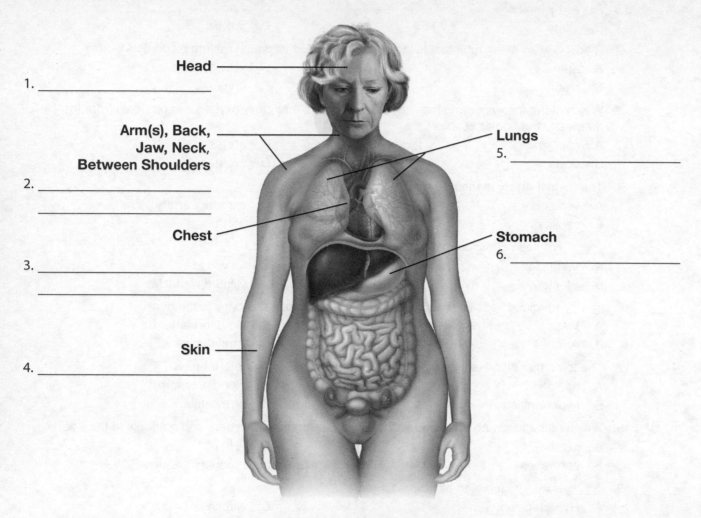

Head ——————

1. _____

**Arm(s), Back,
Jaw, Neck,
Between Shoulders**

2. _____

_____

Chest ——————

3. _____

_____

Skin ——————

4. _____

Lungs

5. _____

Stomach

6. _____

7. In addition to the signs included on this figure, what other symptoms might a person who is having a heart attack experience?

_____

_____

_____

_____

Name _____ Date _____

Cancer Research

In Lesson 14.3, you learned about several common cancers, including skin, lung, breast, and colon cancer. Using reliable online sources, investigate three cancers that were not discussed in detail in your textbook. Obtain the information identified below.

1. Type of cancer: _____

   Online source: _____

   Risk factors for cancer: _____

   _____

   Signs and symptoms: _____

   _____

   Prevention methods: _____

   _____

   Treatment options: _____

   _____

2. Type of cancer: _____

   Online source: _____

   Risk factors for cancer: _____

   _____

   Signs and symptoms: _____

   _____

   Prevention methods: _____

   _____

   Treatment options: _____

   _____

3. Type of cancer: _____

   Online source: _____

   Risk factors for cancer: _____

   _____

   Signs and symptoms: _____

   _____

   Prevention methods: _____

   _____

   Treatment options: _____

   _____

Name _____ Date _____

Signs and Symptoms of Diabetes Mellitus

The major signs and symptoms of diabetes mellitus surface in many of the body's systems. In the figure below, identify the signs and symptoms of diabetes mellitus in each body system.

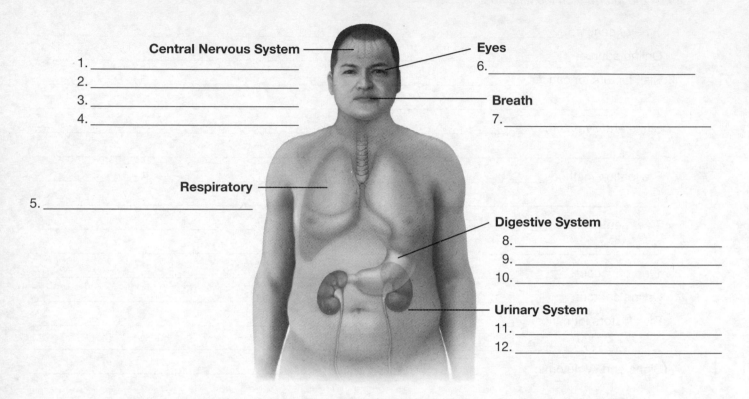

Central Nervous System

1. _____
2. _____
3. _____
4. _____

Eyes

6. _____

Breath

7. _____

Respiratory

5. _____

Digestive System

8. _____
9. _____
10. _____

Urinary System

11. _____
12. _____

13. In addition to the signs included on this figure, what other symptoms might a person who has diabetes mellitus experience?

_____
_____
_____
_____
_____
_____
_____
_____

Chapter 14

Reading Practice

Reread the following passage from the textbook. Then answer the questions that follow.

Cancer is a complex disease, with different forms of the disease having different characteristics. One characteristic that all forms of cancer share is an uncontrolled growth of abnormal cells. All cell reproduction occurs by division of cells, which is the basis for organ growth, tissue repair, and tissue development. Healthy cells control their growth, dividing only when needed. Cancerous cells divide rapidly and produce abnormal cells that do not function like normal cells.

Scientists call a mass of abnormal cells a *tumor*. Tumors fall into two categories. Malignant tumors are cancerous; benign tumors are not.

Benign tumors usually remain in the area of the body where they first develop and do not invade nearby tissues. Moles and skin calluses are examples of benign tumors. Because benign tumors remain localized within organs or tissues, they usually pose few health hazards and may not require treatment. If a benign tumor does cause health problems, it may be more easily removed than a cancerous tumor.

In contrast, *malignant tumors* invade the normal tissues around the area where they first develop. A key characteristic of malignant tumors is *metastasis*. This is the ability to spread to other parts of the body, where additional tumors then develop. Metastasis is possible because malignant cells can break away from the main tumor and enter blood vessels, which transport the malignant cells throughout the body.

_____ 1. Which of the following statements about tumors is accurate?

    A. Both benign and malignant tumors are cancerous.

    B. Benign tumors are cancerous.

    C. Malignant tumors are not cancerous.

    D. Malignant tumors are cancerous.

_____ 2. Why do benign tumors usually pose few health hazards?

    A. They remain small.

    B. They do not grow as fast as malignant tumors.

    C. They remain localized within organs and tissues.

    D. They spread throughout the body.

_____ 3. Which of the following statements correctly describes the process of metastasis?

    A. Malignant cells break away from the main tumor and move through the body via the bloodstream, forming new tumors elsewhere in the body.

    B. Malignant tumors can break off from the area where they first develop and move to a different site in the body.

    C. Benign cells break away from the main tumor and move throughout the body via the bloodstream, forming new tumors elsewhere in the body.

    D. none of the above

Chapter 14

Practice Test

Completion: *Write the term that completes the statement in the space provided.*

1. _____ is the body's internal balance and stability.

2. A sample of tissue removed from the body for microscopic study is called a(n)
   _____.

3. Produced in the pancreas, _____ is a hormone that directs cells to
   consume blood glucose.

4. _____ is a condition characterized by dangerously high blood glucose
   levels.

5. Allergies that affect a specific part of the body are known as _____.

True/False: *Indicate whether each statement below is true or false by circling either T or F.*

T   F   6. Proto-oncogenes turn on cell division as needed.

T   F   7. Relapse is a period of time in which the signs and symptoms of a disease subside.

T   F   8. Veins are blood vessels that carry blood from the heart to the capillaries.

T   F   9. The aorta is the largest vein in the body.

T   F   10. A benign tumor is not cancerous.

Multiple Choice: *Write the letter that corresponds to the correct answer in the blank space.*

_____ 11. _____ is a condition in which the heart is too weak to pump blood effectively.
   A. Atherosclerosis   C. Coronary artery disease
   B. Congestive heart failure   D. Hypertension

_____ 12. Diseases that are noninfectious are also known as _____.
   A. communicable diseases   C. severe diseases
   B. noncommunicable diseases   D. complicated diseases

_____ 13. There are two types of stroke—ischemic stroke and the less common _____.
   A. hemorrhagic stroke   C. transient ischemic attack
   B. warning stroke   D. mini-stroke

_____ 14. Disorders of heart rhythm are called _____.
   A. beating irregularities   C. rhythmic inconsistencies
   B. off beats   D. arrhythmias

_____ 15. Which of the following are risk factors for developing cancer?
   A. carcinogens   C. smoking
   B. diet   D. all of the above

Name _____

Matching: *Match each term to its definition by writing the letter of the term in the space provided.*

_____ 16. an immune response in which the body reacts destructively to a harmless substance

_____ 17. a disease in which the body is unable to regulate its levels of glucose

_____ 18. a condition in which the joints become inflamed, causing pain and stiffness

_____ 19. the probable consequence of a disease

_____ 20. allergies that affect the entire body

_____ 21. an allergic response in which fluid fills the lungs and air passages narrow

_____ 22. a substance that causes blood vessels to leak fluids into body tissues, resulting in swelling

A.   prognosis

B.   diabetes mellitus

C.   allergy

D   histamine

E.   arthritis

F.   anaphylaxis

G.   systemic allergies

Analyzing Data: *Use the information provided to answer the following questions.*

Five-Year Relative Survival for Colorectal Cancer

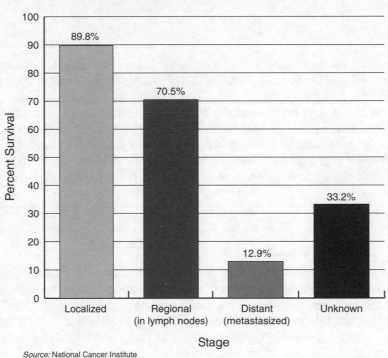

Source: National Cancer Institute

23. Which stage of colorectal cancer has the highest survival rate?

_____

24. Assuming this table represents survival rates for 100 patients, how many more patients with localized stage colorectal cancer survive than patients with distant stage?

_____

Short Answer: *On a separate sheet of paper, answer the following questions using what you have learned in this chapter.*

25. How are communicable and noncommunicable diseases different?

26. Explain the difference between type 1 diabetes mellitus and type 2 diabetes mellitus.

Lesson 15.1

Emotional Intelligence

EQ, or emotional (intelligence) quotient, is a measurement of one's skill at identifying and evaluating emotions and at expressing emotions in healthy, positive ways. Analyze each scenario presented below and indicate how the participants could have been more emotionally intelligent.

1. Since Reagan began dating Kelsey, Reagan's friends rarely get to spend time with her. They all used to eat lunch together in the high school cafeteria; now Reagan usually leaves school to go out for lunch with Kelsey. What's more, Reagan rarely replies to her friends' text messages. One afternoon, Sara, one of Reagan's longtime friends, confronts her in the locker room after gym class. "What is up with you and Kelsey?" she snaps. "Aren't we good enough to hang out with you anymore?" How do you think Sara could have transformed her negative-EQ response to this situation into a positive one?

   _____

   _____

   _____

2. Stephen has a sarcastic sense of humor and sometimes hurts other people's feelings. He often does impressions of teachers and classmates, which his friends think are hilarious and spot-on. One morning before the bell has rung, Stephen is immersed in a scathingly animated impression of his classmate Jon. When Jon enters the classroom, he notices the other students crowded in a circle around Stephen; they are rapt with attention. Jon realizes what is happening as one of the other students quickly motions to Stephen to stop doing his impression. Stephen turns to see Jon walking toward his desk in the back of the room. "Hey, I was only joking," Stephen says dismissively. Jon, sulking, ignores him. How do you think both Stephen and Jon could have transformed their negative-EQ responses to this situation into positive ones?

   _____

   _____

   _____

3. Aisha, a new student at Kennedy High School, has begun to date Alec. Aisha is unaware that Alec recently broke up with Rhiannon, his girlfriend of more than a year. One afternoon during lunch, Rhiannon approaches Aisha and tells her that Alec is bad news and he eventually will "dump" Aisha. Later, Aisha learns that Rhiannon is still hurt and angry because Alec broke up with her. How do you think Rhiannon could have transformed her negative-EQ responses to this situation into a positive one?

   _____

   _____

   _____

4. Bob and Paul are high school seniors competing for a part-time internship at a prestigious law firm. Bob has worked hard, earning mostly As in his coursework on top of caring for his younger sister with Down syndrome. Paul has maintained a B-minus average and has a reputation for being the class clown. Shortly after their interviews, Bob is astonished to learn that Paul was selected for the internship. Bob cannot bring himself to congratulate his rival. Instead, he remarks to Paul that "apparently slackers are 'in' this year." How do you think Bob could have transformed his negative-EQ responses to this situation into a positive one?

   _____

   _____

   _____

Name _____ Date _____

What's Your EQ?

Your EQ, or emotional (intelligence) quotient, is a measurement of how well you identify and evaluate emotions, and of how well you express your emotion. For this activity, write about a time that you demonstrated emotional intelligence or, upon reflection, did not express it as well as you wish you had.

1. Describe the situation. What happened? How did the other person or people involved in the situation act? How did you act? If you were to have a similar experience today, what would you do or say differently?

_____

_____

_____

_____

_____

_____

_____

_____

_____

_____

_____

_____

_____

2. How important is emotional intelligence in comparison to intellectual intelligence? Explain your answer.

_____

_____

_____

_____

_____

_____

_____

_____

Name _____ Date _____

Key Concepts Review

Multiple Choice: *Write the letter that corresponds to the correct answer in the blank space.*

_____ 1. Which of the following elements contribute(s) to personal identity?
   A. physical identity
   B. active identity
   C. passive identity
   D. both A and B

_____ 2. Which of the following definitions best describes the concept of *core values*?
   A. a basic understanding of the concepts of good and evil
   B. tolerance for cultural and personal differences in belief systems
   C. the fundamental beliefs and ideals that people have about the attitudes they hold and how they want to act
   D. the intersection of self-exploration and self-knowledge

_____ 3. Which term is defined as "possessing characteristics of both sexes"?
   A. androgenic
   B. androgynous
   C. androgynoid
   D. synandrogenic

_____ 4. Which of the following could be a role model?
   A. parent
   B. celebrity
   C. historical figure
   D. all of the above

_____ 5. _____ is an expression of how an individual feels about and expresses his or her gender.
   A. Gender identity
   B. Gender role
   C. Gender ideal
   D. Gender stereotype

_____ 6. Which of the following is *not* a stage in the development of ethnic identity?
   A. unexamined/diffused ethnic identity
   B. incremental assimilation
   C. identity search/moratorium
   D. achievement/secure sense of identity

_____ 7. Which of the following statements expresses a gender stereotype?
   A. Teenage girls are emotional.
   B. Teenage girls should have opportunities to play the same sports that teenage boys do.
   C. Teenage boys should be masculine.
   D. both A and C

True/False: *Indicate whether each statement below is true or false by circling either T or F.*

T   F   8. Gender identity is limited to biological makeup—that is, whether a person is female or male.

T   F   9. According to Erik Erikson, teenagers who struggle to develop a sense of personal identity are experiencing *role confusion*.

T   F   10. Gender roles are roles that a person embraces as a result of external expectations and pressures.

T   F   11. A gender stereotype is a behavior or attitude that a society considers "appropriate" for males or females.

T   F   12. A person who is described as *androgynous* is perceived to have masculine and feminine characteristics.

Lesson 15.2

Gender Stereotypes

In a 2008 Pew Research Center survey, 1,190 women and 1,060 men in the United States were asked to identify positive and negative leadership traits, and to indicate whether these traits are more characteristic of men or women. The results of the survey appear in the chart below. The "Total" row beneath each character trait represents the mean percentage (average). Review the chart and answer the questions that follow.

Traits of Men and Women			
Is this characteristic more true of...	**Men** %	**Women** %	**Both, equally** %
Decisive			
Total respondents	44	33	18
Male respondents	48	29	19
Female respondents	40	37	17
Ambitious			
Total respondents	34	34	29
Male respondents	40	27	30
Female respondents	29	39	28
Manipulative			
Total respondents	26	52	16
Male respondents	21	57	16
Female respondents	32	48	16
Intelligent			
Total respondents	14	38	43
Male respondents	18	33	43
Female respondents	10	43	43
Creative			
Total respondents	11	62	24
Male respondents	14	54	28
Female respondents	8	68	20
Compassionate			
Total respondents	5	80	13
Male respondents	7	78	14
Female respondents	3	83	12
Emotional			
Total respondents	5	85	9
Male respondents	7	83	9
Female respondents	3	87	9

1. On a scale of 1–10 (with 10 being the highest and 1 being the lowest), rate *yourself* on the character traits represented in this graph. Explain your answers.

_____

Explanation: _____

_____

Explanation: _____

_____

Explanation: _____

_____

Explanation: _____

_____

Explanation: _____

_____

Explanation: _____

_____

Explanation: _____

Source: Pew Research Center: "Men or Women: Who's the Better Leader? A Paradox in Public Attitudes." August 25, 2008. URL: http://www.pewsocialtrends.org/2008/08/25/men-or-women-whos-the-better-leader/. Accessed October 6, 2014.

(Continued)

2. What percentage of male respondents regard women as the more "creative" sex? Do you think this perception is true or untrue? Explain your answer.

_____

_____

_____

_____

_____

3. How do men and women view themselves with regard to ambition? What do their responses reveal?

_____

_____

_____

_____

_____

4. Seventy-eight percent of men believe women are more compassionate than men, whereas eighty-three percent of women believe they are more compassionate than men. What social factors do you think account for these perceptions? Explain your answer.

_____

_____

_____

_____

_____

5. On which character traits do men give themselves lower ratings than they give women? On which traits do women give themselves lower ratings than they give men? What can you conclude about the disparity in their perceptions? Explain your answer.

_____

_____

_____

_____

_____

6. According to the chart in this activity, what traits do male and female respondents consider to be most characteristic of their genders? What can you conclude about their responses?

_____

_____

_____

_____

_____

Chapter 15

Reading Practice

Reread the following passage from the textbook. Then answer the questions on the next page.

Maslow's Hierarchy of Human Needs

How do you reach your full potential? According to Maslow, achieving self-actualization occurs only after you meet your basic needs. People strive to meet different types of needs after their basic needs are met.

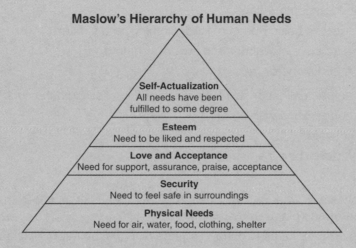

Maslow's Hierarchy of Human Needs

At the most basic level, people must be able to meet their physical needs for survival. These needs include having food to eat, water to drink, and shelter from extreme cold and extreme heat. Once the basic physical needs are met, people work on meeting the needs listed in the next level. People need to feel secure or safe in their surroundings, including home, school, and work environments.

The next level of Maslow's hierarchy focuses on the need for love and acceptance. This need includes feeling connected with friends and family members and having emotional support from those around you.

The fourth level of Maslow's hierarchy focuses on the individual, and particularly on a person's need to feel good about himself or herself. People also have a need for respect from those around them and a need to feel good about themselves.

Finally, the highest level of needs is the need for self-actualization—the need to reach your full potential. People who are self-actualized continually strive to do everything they are capable of doing. They are focused on continuing to grow, learn, and develop throughout their lives to be the best they can be.

Achieving Self-Actualization

People who are achieving self-actualization and reaching their full potential share certain characteristics. These include

- accepting themselves and others for who they are;
- feeling self-motivated instead of relying on other people to provide motivation;
- working actively to solve problems in the world and in their community, including taking responsibility for finding solutions and helping other people to resolve problems;
- viewing the world with a sense of appreciation, inspiration, and pleasure;
- enjoying spending time with other people, but also feeling a need for independence and time alone; and
- feeling at peace with themselves and the world.

(Continued)

_____ 1. Which of the following best embodies the definition of *self-actualization*?

    A. the fulfillment of one's basic needs

    B. the need for reassurance from others

    C. the realization of one's full potential

    D. development of an appropriately cautious view of the world

_____ 2. What is the second level of Maslow's hierarchy of needs?

    A. the need to feel safe in one's surroundings

    B. the need for support, assurance, praise, and acceptance

    C. the need to be liked and respected

    D. the need for air, water, food, clothing, and shelter

_____ 3. Which of the following would *not* be considered self-actualization?

    A. producing a documentary film

    B. striving to meet the basic needs of food, clothing, and shelter

    C. experiencing a sense of wonder and awe over nature

    D. completing a 26-kilometer race

_____ 4. The process of self-actualization involves which of the following behaviors?

    A. developing connections with others

    B. being self-motivated

    C. feeling comfortable being alone

    D. all of the above

_____ 5. Based on this passage, what can you infer about the needs of an impoverished family living in an inner-city neighborhood plagued by violent crime?

    A. The family's primary focus is on fulfilling needs in the top tier of Maslow's hierarchy.

    B. The family's primary focus is on fulfilling needs in level one of Maslow's hierarchy.

    C. The family's primary focus is on fulfilling needs in level two of Maslow's hierarchy.

    D. both B and C

_____ 6. Which statement best expresses the main idea of this passage?

    A. Believing that you are living up to your full potential—or achieving self-actualization—is an important part of feeling good about yourself.

    B. People who are self-actualized continually strive to do everything they are capable of doing.

    C. Once basic physical needs are met, people can work on meeting the needs listed in the next level of Maslow's hierarchy.

    D. The need for independence and the need to spend time alone are crucial to achieving self-actualization.

Chapter 15

Practice Test

Completion: *Write the term that completes the statement in the space provided.*

1. People who have a positive outlook on life, and therefore seem better able to cope with difficulties, have _____.

2. The ability to recover from stressful and traumatic events is called _____.

3. _____ is the ability to imagine yourself in someone else's place, and to understand someone else's wants, needs, and point of view.

4. The ability to control one's emotions and impulses and to act with careful deliberation and integrity is called _____.

5. _____ are culturally defined assumptions about what it means to be male or female.

True/False: *Indicate whether each statement below is true or false by circling either T or F.*

T   F   6. People with high emotional intelligence are skilled at understanding the emotions that other people are feeling.

T   F   7. Social identity is defined as one's engagement in particular activities and interests, such as science, music, sports, and community service.

T   F   8. The belief that only boys should play football is an example of a gender stereotype.

T   F   9. An American teenager who speaks a Celtic language, participates in Irish dancing competitions, and annually visits Ireland with her family has a strong sense of ethnicity.

T   F   10. According to Erikson, people develop either a sense of personal identity or confusion about identity between 12 and 18 years of age.

Multiple Choice: *Write the letter that corresponds to the correct answer in the blank space.*

_____ 11. Which of the following factors affect(s) self-esteem?

    A. home, school, community, and cultural environments

    B. social interactions with family members, friends, and others

    C. media, such as television, movies, and social networking sites

    D. all of the above

_____ 12. _____ is the status of a person who is entitled to the rights and duties of a community.

    A. Philanthropy

    B. Citizenship

    C. Ethnicity

    D. both B and C

_____ 13. A philanthropist is an individual who _____.

    A. has the rights and duties of all members of a community

    B. has a zest for life

    C. is philosophical

    D. makes donations to improve others' lives and well-being

_____ 14. Which of the following is *not* a strategy for improving intellectual health?

    A. evaluating decisions after you have executed them

    B. developing a new skill or interest

    C. playing games that strengthen your knowledge, creativity, or problem-solving skills

    D. none of the above

(Continued)

_____ 15. In the top tier of Maslow's hierarchy, people are concerned with which of the following?

    A. meeting basic needs (water, food, clothing, shelter)

    B. feeling safe in their environment

    C. achieving self-actualization

    D. feeling accepted by others

Matching: *Match each key term to its definition by writing the corresponding letter in the space provided.*

_____ 16. who you are, including your physical traits, activities, social connections, and internal thoughts and feelings

_____ 17. a person's biological makeup—male or female—and how a person experiences or expresses that makeup

_____ 18. your mental picture of yourself

_____ 19. the act of thinking repeatedly about something for a long period of time; a habit of negative thinking that can trigger anxiety and depression

_____ 20. the ability to identify one's own emotions and understand the emotions of others

_____ 21. your feelings of self-worth

_____ 22. the ability to maintain a positive outlook in the face of challenge, hardship, and change

_____ 23. the feeling that you are striving toward and becoming the best person you can be

_____ 24. a person's connection to a cultural or national social group

_____ 25. culturally defined assumptions about what it means to be male or female

_____ 26. attitudes and behaviors that a society considers "appropriate" for males or females

_____ 27. a person who makes charitable donations to help improve other people's well-being

_____ 28. the status of a person who is recognized by the laws of a state or country as having the rights and duties of all members of a community

_____ 29. the ability to imagine yourself in someone else's place, and to understand someone else's wants, needs, and point of view

_____ 30. term that refers to people who exhibit feminine and masculine traits equally

A. androgynous

B. citizenship

C. emotional intelligence

D. empathy

E. ethnicity

F. gender identity

G. gender roles

H. gender stereotypes

I. identity

J. optimism

K. philanthropist

L. rumination

M. self-actualization

N. self-esteem

O. self-image

Student Challenge: *Working in small groups, select one of the topics below. Research the topic (the Pew Research Center website is a good place to begin) and prepare a report, along with questions to stimulate class discussion. Share your report with the rest of the class.*

A. What gender stereotypes exist in your generation? How do those stereotypes compare to the stereotypes in past generations? Cite specific studies and statistics and present your answers.

B. In your generation, is there a gap between the amount of men who hold bachelor's degrees and the amount of women? Cite specific studies and statistics and present your answers.

C. Does a wage gap between genders still exist in your generation? Cite specific studies and statistics and present your answers.

D. What are women's and men's views on gender and work in your generation? Are women discouraged from working outside the home? How common are stay-at-home fathers? Cite specific studies and statistics and present your answers.

E. How do families divide home responsibilities in your generation? Does gender affect this division of responsibilities? Cite specific studies and statistics and present your answers.

Lesson 16.1

Acute versus Chronic Stress

You will encounter various stressors throughout your life. Some will be acute (short-lived), while others will be chronic (long-lasting). For this activity, review the stressors in the table below. Then, categorize the stressors as either acute or chronic. Finally, complete the table by adding five stressors you have experienced in your own life. Identify whether these stressors are acute or chronic.

Stressor	Acute	Chronic
1. Your family is moving to a new state next week.		
2. Your Spanish teacher has assigned an important project, but only gives you four days to complete it.		
3. It is 10:00 p.m. on the night before your biology final, and you don't feel prepared.		
4. Your mother announces that she's pregnant.		
5. You realize your sister took your favorite jeans.		
6. Your best friend tagged an embarrassing picture of you online.		
7. Your parents announce they are getting a divorce.		
8. You accidentally respond to a group text with a message meant only for your best friend.		
9. You are waiting in the lobby of a potential employer before for your first job interview.		
10. Your grandmother is diagnosed with breast cancer.		
11.		
12.		
13.		
14.		
15.		

Lesson 16.1

The Most Stressful Cities in the US

In chapter 16's Local and Global Health feature, "Are Some Countries More Stressful Than Others?", you learned that people in some countries report higher satisfaction and less stress than people in other countries. Several studies have explored the idea that some US cities are more stressful than others. Find one of these studies online and choose three cities that are considered to be the most stressful. Then, identify the stressors that residents of each city face. Finally, identify stressors in your own hometown and describe how your hometown compares to the cities on this list.

Title of study: _____

Web source: _____

1. City #1: _____

   Stress ranking: _____

   Stressors: _____

   _____

2. City #2: _____

   Stress ranking: _____

   Stressors: _____

   _____

3. City #3: _____

   Stress ranking: _____

   Stressors: _____

   _____

4. Your hometown: _____

   Stressors: _____

   _____

How does your hometown compare to other cities on the list? Is it as stressful? less stressful? Explain your response.

_____

_____

_____

_____

Lesson 16.2

Physical Responses to Stress

Physical responses to stress vary among people. How you respond to stress might not be how your friend or family member responds to stress. For this activity, choose one stressful event that you and one of your family members have both experienced. Record your physical response to this stressful event on the lines below. Then, ask a family member how his or her body responded to this stressful event. Record the response and compare your results.

Stressful event: _____

Your physical response:

_____

_____

_____

_____

_____

_____

_____

Family member's physical response:

_____

_____

_____

_____

_____

_____

How do you and your family member's physical responses compare? Do your bodies respond to stress in the same way, or were your responses quite different? Explain your answers.

_____

_____

_____

_____

_____

_____

Lesson 16.3

Intellectual and Emotional Effects of Stress

Stress affects your physical health, but it also has an impact on your intellectual and emotional health. The following scenarios describe teenagers who are experiencing various stressors in their lives. Read the scenarios below and then identify the intellectual and emotional side effects each individual may be experiencing as a result of stress. Finally, describe how each individual might manage his or her stress well.

1. Jaden and his family recently moved across town. While Jaden loves their new house, he now has to attend a different high school for his senior year. He wishes his parents would have waited until he had graduated high school to move. At his old school, Jaden was captain of the basketball team and had lots of friends. Jaden plans on joining the basketball team at his new school, but is worried this coach won't give him as much playing time as he had on his previous team. He's also finding it hard both to make friends at his new school and to spend time with his old friends. What intellectual and emotional side effects might stress have on Jaden? What can he do to manage this stress well?

    _____

    _____

    _____

    _____

    _____

    _____

2. Maya is supposed to take the SAT on Friday. This will be her second time taking the test. The first time she took it, her score did not meet admissions requirements for the college she wants to attend. Maya hopes that by studying and taking practice exams, she will do much better this time. Unfortunately, it seems like every time she sits down to study, her younger brother and sister interrupt her. What intellectual and emotional side effects might stress have on Maya? What can she do to manage this stress well?

    _____

    _____

    _____

    _____

    _____

3. Will and Tina have been dating for most of their freshman year. Last week, Tina told Will she thinks they should just be friends. The two share a lot of friends, and Will is afraid Tina's friends will stop being friends with him now that he and Tina are no longer together. They are also in the same algebra, history, and French classes, and he worries those classes will be hard to sit through. What intellectual and emotional side effects might stress have on Will? What can he do to manage this stress well?

    _____

    _____

    _____

    _____

    _____

Lesson 16.4

How Would You Handle It?

All people respond to stress in different ways. For this activity, read the following scenarios describing fictional teens and their stressors. Then, decide how you would handle the stress each individual is facing. Write your stress-management plan for each stressor in the spaces provided.

1. Last month, Shana's parents announced they are getting a divorce. Shana was taken completely by surprise—she had never even seen them fight! Since her dad moved out, Shana's mom has been crying a lot, and Shana feels guilty for going out with friends and leaving her mom alone. How would you handle the stress Shana is facing? Describe your stress-management plan.

   _____

   _____

   _____

   _____

2. Miguel has always been involved in a lot of school activities. He's on the wrestling team, participates in HOSA competitions, and is a peer advisor at his school. Last month, Miguel's parents told him they cannot afford to help pay for his college education. Miguel decided he would get a part-time job at the local car wash to help save money for school. In addition to school and extracurricular activities, Miguel is now working 15 hours a week. His schoolwork is starting to suffer, he's tired all the time, and last week he forgot about a peer-advisor meeting he was supposed to attend. How would you handle the stress Miguel is facing? Describe your stress-management plan.

   _____

   _____

   _____

   _____

3. After Lena's mom, Cindy, married her boyfriend, Dave, Lena and Cindy moved into Dave's house. The house is twenty minutes away from the town where Lena used to live and she had to switch schools in the middle of the year. Now, Cindy and Dave have announced they're having a baby. Lena feels left out and misses her old friends. How would you handle the stress Lena is facing? Describe your stress-management plan.

   _____

   _____

   _____

   _____

4. Until last week when she broke her wrist at volleyball practice, Claire had been a starter on the team. Not being able to play has left Claire irritable, not to mention she feels like she has tons of energy to burn. How would you handle the stress Claire is facing? Describe your stress-management plan.

   _____

   _____

   _____

   _____

Chapter 16

Reading Practice

Reread the following passage from the textbook. Then answer the questions that follow.

Stress and Body Systems

Stress impacts different body systems, which can then lead to many health problems. Body systems particularly affected by stress include the nervous, endocrine, cardiovascular, immune, and reproductive systems.

The Nervous System

The nervous system consists of the brain, the spinal cord, and the neural pathways that bring information to and from the brain. This body system sends messages to the brain that your body is receiving particular sensations—such as touch and pain. The nervous system is responsible for mobilizing your body to react to a threatening situation because it regulates many other body systems. In the face of a threat, your nervous system prompts various body systems to act. These systems increase respiration and heart rate, decrease digestion and reproduction, and send blood to the muscles. These physiological changes improve your body's ability to respond to threatening situations.

The Endocrine System

The endocrine system is a set of glands that release hormones into the bloodstream. These hormones then travel though the bloodstream to cause changes in a particular body tissue or organ. During times of stress, the central nervous system stimulates the endocrine glands to secrete *epinephrine* and *norepinephrine*, which are known as the **stress hormones**. These hormones trigger the physiological effects that help the body respond quickly to a threat.

_____ 1. Body systems that are particularly affected by stress include the nervous, endocrine, cardiovascular, immune, and _____ systems.
   A. integumentary
   B. skeletal
   C. urinary
   D. reproductive

_____ 2. The endocrine system is comprised of _____.
   A. muscles
   B. glands
   C. neural pathways
   D. lymph nodes

_____ 3. What are stress hormones?
   A. hormones that trigger the body's physiological response to stress
   B. hormones that cause stress
   C. epinephrine and norepinephrine
   D. both A and C

Chapter 16

Practice Test

Completion: *Write the term that completes the statement in the space provided.*

1. When stress continues over long periods of time, it is known as _____.

2. Your body's response to stress can be divided into three stages: alarm stage, _____, and exhaustion stage.

3. The body's _____ system defends against infection and disease.

4. _____ is a mood or emotional state characterized by feelings of low self-worth and a lack of interest in daily life activities.

5. PTSD stands for _____.

True/False: *Indicate whether each statement below is true or false by circling either T or F.*

T F 6. School is the only source of stress for teenagers.

T F 7. Stress does not affect a person's physical health.

T F 8. People who experience chronic stress are at a greater risk for developing cancer.

T F 9. Stress can affect a person's intellectual and emotional health.

T F 10. Well-managed stress can be used to your benefit.

Multiple Choice: *Write the letter that corresponds to the correct answer in the blank space.*

_____ 11. High levels of stress are associated with which of the following unhealthy lifestyle choices?
   A. smoking cigarettes
   B. using alcohol or drugs
   C. eating fewer vegetables
   D. all of the above

_____ 12. Which of the following relaxation techniques can be used to change how your body responds to stress?
   A. yoga
   B. meditation
   C. writing in a journal
   D. both A and B

_____ 13. Which of the following is a function of the nervous system?
   A. defending against infection and disease
   B. producing hormones
   C. pumping blood throughout the body
   D. initiating the fight-or-flight response

_____ 14. Which of the following is an example of acute stress?
   A. A parent loses his or her job.
   B. Your parents separate.
   C. You have been fighting with your sister nearly every day.
   D. Your English paper is due tomorrow.

_____ 15. The _____ is the part of the brain involved in the formation and storage of memory.
   A. pons
   B. medulla oblongata
   C. hippocampus
   D. hypothalamus

(Continued)

Name _____ Date _____

Matching: *Match each term to its definition by writing the letter of the term in the space provided.*

_____ 16. the strategy of focusing on the positive aspects of a stressful event

_____ 17. the strategy of imagining a pleasant environment when faced with stress

_____ 18. white blood cells that eliminate or disable foreign and possible infected cells

_____ 19. the strategy of tensing and then relaxing each part of your body and breathing deeply to relieve stress

_____ 20. term for the body's physical and psychological response to traumatic or challenging situations

_____ 21. disagreements or problems that result from opposing actions or views

_____ 22. the strategy of clearing negative thoughts from your mind and relaxing your body to relieve stress

_____ 23. the capacity to think and reason

A. lymphocytes

B. meditation

C. progressive muscle relaxation

D. positive reappraisal

E. visualization

F. conflicts

G. cognitive ability

H. stress

Analyzing Data: *Use the information provided to answer the following questions.*

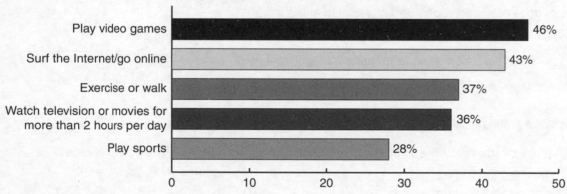

Stress-Management Techniques of Teens

Play video games — 46%
Surf the Internet/go online — 43%
Exercise or walk — 37%
Watch television or movies for more than 2 hours per day — 36%
Play sports — 28%

Source: American Psychological Association

24. Assuming 100 students responded to the survey, how many more students watch television or a movie to relieve stress than play a sport?

_____

_____

25. Identify two stress-management techniques that are not included in the graph above.

_____

_____

Short Answer: *On a separate sheet of paper, answer the following questions using what you have learned in this chapter.*

26. How might stress cause physical exhaustion?

27. Why is it wise to avoid using tobacco, alcohol, and drugs, particularly when experiencing stress?

Lesson 17.1

Key Terms Review

Matching: *Match each key term to its definition by writing the letter of the term in the space provided.*

_____ 1. a medical condition in which a person experiences mental or emotional problems that are severe or persistent enough to interfere with daily functioning

_____ 2. a mental illness characterized by delusions, hallucinations, and irregular thought patterns

_____ 3. episodes of intense fear that are often accompanied by serious physical symptoms

_____ 4. a mental illness characterized by a person's extreme instability in his or her self-concept and relationships

_____ 5. a mental illness characterized by intense periods of depression closely followed by extreme positive, or manic feelings

_____ 6. a mental illness characterized by extreme or unrealistic worries about daily events, experiences, or objects

_____ 7. a common mental illness characterized by disregard for social rules, a tendency for impulsive behavior, and indifference toward other people

_____ 8. a mental illness characterized by intense and ongoing negative feelings such as hopelessness, sadness, or loneliness

A. antisocial personality disorder

B. anxiety disorder

C. bipolar disorder

D. borderline personality disorder

E. major depression

F. mental illness

G. panic attacks

H. schizophrenia

Short Answer: *Using all of the key terms covered in this review, write one or two paragraphs explaining how the key terms relate to one another and to their definitions.*

_____

_____

_____

_____

_____

_____

_____

_____

_____

_____

_____

_____

_____

_____

Lesson 17.1

Identifying Mental Illnesses and Disorders

A mental illness is a medical condition in which a person experiences a mental or emotional problem that is severe enough to interfere with daily life. Each mental illness, or mental disorder, has its own set of symptoms that affect daily functioning. In each of the following scenarios, the person described is experiencing a mental illness or disorder. Read each of the scenarios and determine which mental illness or disorder he or she has. Then, explain how that mental illness or disorder might affect the person's daily functioning.

1. Jim is at a concert with his friends. He was so excited to get tickets that he didn't have time to think about the large crowd he would encounter. Halfway through the concert, Jim begins to feel that something bad might happen. There are so many people in the concert hall, and the music seems to be getting louder. Jim is nauseous and he can feel his heart racing. What mental illness or disorder is Jim experiencing? How does this affect his daily functioning?

   _____

   _____

   _____

   _____

2. Last year, Kate was sexually assaulted. For weeks after the incident, Kate was afraid of nearly everything. She was unable to return to school for about a month. Although she has improved and returned to school, Kate still feels nervous and afraid sometimes, even though she is no longer in danger. Kate cannot seem to stop thinking about the assault. What mental illness or disorder is Kate experiencing? How does this affect her daily functioning?

   _____

   _____

   _____

   _____

3. Corey, a freshman, is finding the transition to high school difficult. He can't seem to pay attention in class, and he feels bored doing class assignments and activities. He forgets instructions the teacher gives, and often does assignments the wrong way as a result. What mental illness or disorder is Corey experiencing? How does this affect his daily functioning?

   _____

   _____

   _____

   _____

4. Shannon's best friend, Cara, is acting strangely. Cara has been anxious in class and turns down invitations to hang out. One day, Shannon glimpses small cuts on Cara's arm. When Shannon asks Cara about it, Cara says it's nothing, but Shannon is worried. What mental illness or disorder is Cara experiencing? How does this affect her daily functioning?

   _____

   _____

   _____

   _____

Lesson 17.2

Which Factor?

In most cases, the cause of a mental illness or disorder is unknown. However, scientists believe that several factors—including genetics, brain injury, environment, and cognitive distortions—contribute to the development of these disorders. Read each of the scenarios below and determine what factors may be causing each person's mental illness or disorder.

1. Tim is a star on his high school football team. He plays in almost every game and has received awards for his performance on the field. Playing football can be dangerous, though, and Tim has had several concussions in his time on the team. The last time he got a concussion, Tim acted strangely afterward. He was anxious and even lashed out angrily at his friends and girlfriend when they offered their help.

   _____

   _____

   _____

   _____

   _____

2. Recently, Malia's parents got divorced. At first, Malia thought she was okay with this because her parents used to fight a lot. However, the stress of shuttling between her mom's and dad's house has started to affect her. She feels anxious at school, has trouble finishing assignments, and is having obsessive-compulsive urges.

   _____

   _____

   _____

   _____

   _____

3. Frankie is a straight-A student, but he often has low self-esteem. When he has trouble completing an assignment or doesn't get the right answer on his first try, Frankie's immediate thought is, "I am a failure." No matter what his friends and family tell him, he cannot seem to shake the thought.

   _____

   _____

   _____

   _____

   _____

4. For as long as Dana can remember, her mother has been a very sad person. Sometimes her mom would spend days in her bedroom and would not talk to anyone. Now, Dana realizes her mother has depression. Dana has begun to experience the same symptoms.

   _____

   _____

   _____

   _____

   _____

Lesson 17.2

Recognizing Cognitive Distortions

Cognitive distortions are unhealthy patterns of thinking that people have about the world around them. These patterns of thinking can easily lead to mental illness or disorder. People can correct these distortions, but they first need to recognize them. Study the list of distortions below and then match each scenario with the distortion that is being experienced.

Distortions

A. black-and-white thinking

B. jumping to conclusions

C. catastrophizing

D. control fallacies

E. emotional reasoning

F. fallacy of change

G. always being right

Scenarios

_____ 1. Kim is a straight-A student, but when she gets a bad grade on one exam, she is convinced she won't be able to get into college.

_____ 2. Bob does not often take time to relax. One week, he decides to allow himself a lazy weekend and spends the two days watching television. On Sunday evening, Bob feels worried that he will always be this lazy.

_____ 3. Gerald is an average student, but he often thinks about himself in extremes. If he does well on a test, he thinks, "I am perfect!" But if he does badly on a test, he thinks, "I am a failure!"

_____ 4. Pearl's boyfriend, John, is not as neat as she is and doesn't care about grades as much as she does. She knows this when she begins dating him and intends to make him change.

_____ 5. Stephanie is a naturally shy person. When she meets new people, she does not speak with them right away. This often leads people to think that she is stuck-up or doesn't like them.

_____ 6. When Andrew argues with people, he has one goal in mind: winning. Instead of listening to what the other person has to say, he concentrates on what his next response will be.

_____ 7. Mallory gets a bad grade on her English paper. Although she spent most of the week watching TV and working on other assignments, Mallory blames the teacher for her bad grade. "She didn't give us enough time," Mallory says.

Lesson 17.3

Suicide Prevention

Suicide is one of the leading causes of death among teenagers and young adults in the United States. It can be difficult to predict who may attempt suicide, but there are certain signs that can indicate someone may be considering it. If you recognize any of these warning signs in someone you love, there are steps that you can take.

Review the warning signs of suicide that are covered in your textbook. Then, in the following situations, identify which warning signs are present. Finally, give concrete examples of what you could do to prevent the potential suicide.

1. Your friend Sasha has been missing book club meetings. She used to love going to book club and often engaged in passionate discussions about the group's recent read. When you ask her about it, Sasha shrugs and says she hasn't been feeling up to attending the meetings. You find out from another friend of Sasha's that she has been missing her tennis lessons as well. You also notice that Sasha has been absent from social media lately. What warning signs is Sasha is exhibiting? What could you do to help prevent her potential suicide?

   _____

   _____

   _____

   _____

2. One day, your friend Caleb unexpectedly gives you his guitar. He saved up for two summers to buy that guitar and often said that it was his most treasured possession. A few days later, your friend Jenny says that Caleb gave away his favorite video game console and a large portion of his book collection. What warning signs is Caleb is exhibiting? What could you do to help prevent his potential suicide?

   _____

   _____

   _____

   _____

3. Michelle used to be your happiest, most upbeat friend. When you were feeling down, her infectious good attitude could always cheer you up. She was the chatterbox of your group of friends, always ready to talk your ear off. Recently, however, Michelle has not been acting like herself. She has been broody and seems caught up in her own thoughts. When you asked her what was wrong, Michelle simply shrugged and continued scribbling in a notebook. What warning signs is Michelle exhibiting? What could you do to help prevent her potential suicide?

   _____

   _____

   _____

   _____

Lesson 17.4

Finding Reliable Health Information

For this activity, you will find three sources of reliable information for each of the three topics listed below. You may use the sources of information given in Figure 1.6, "Health and Safety Information," or you may research your own sources. For each source, write the name of the organization and the title of the article or web page. If the source does not appear in Figure 1.6, list its website address as well. Do not use a source more than once.

Topic: *Therapy for mental illnesses and disorders*

1. A. Website #1 (name of organization) _____

   B. Title of article or web page _____

2. A. Website #2 (name of organization) _____

   B. Title of article or web page _____

3. A. Website #3 (name of organization) _____

   B. Title of article or web page _____

Topic: *Social stigma surrounding mental illnesses and disorders*

1. A. Website #1 (name of organization) _____

   B. Title of article or web page _____

2. A. Website #2 (name of organization) _____

   B. Title of article or web page _____

3. A. Website #3 (name of organization) _____

   B. Title of article or web page _____

Topic: *Medication used to treat mental illnesses and disorders*

1. A. Website #1 (name of organization) _____

   B. Title of article or web page _____

2. A. Website #2 (name of organization) _____

   B. Title of article or web page _____

3. A. Webslte #3 (name of organization) _____

   B. Title of article or web page _____

After compiling the above information about your sources, answer the following questions:

1. Of the three sources you chose for each topic, which sources were most reliable? How do you know?

_____

_____

2. Which sources provided the most interesting information? Write three facts you learned about each topic.

_____

_____

Lesson 17.4

Mental Health Careers

In the Spotlight on Health and Wellness Careers feature in this chapter, several careers that relate to mental health are discussed. When choosing a healthcare career, you should be mindful of your personal interests, strengths, and weaknesses. These will help you decide which career would best suit you. Study the chart below, which is organized according to interest or personal quality, and then answer the questions on the next page. Keep in mind your own interests, strengths, and weaknesses when reviewing the chart.

Interest/Quality	Career	Duties	Education and Training	Resources
An interest in science	Psychiatrist	Diagnoses mental illnesses and disorders	Bachelor's degree, medical degree, certification exam	American Psychiatric Association
	Psychiatric nurse	Tests patients to learn symptoms and patterns of illness	Nursing degree, specialized training in psychiatry and psychotherapy, direct clinical training	American Psychiatric Nurses Association
Enjoys working with people	Psychologist	Provides psychotherapy directly to patients	Doctoral degree, licensing exam	Society of Clinical Psychology, American Psychological Association
	Clinical social worker	Treats patients directly for mental, behavioral, and emotional issues	Master's degree, supervised clinical therapy	National Association of Social Workers
	Marriage and family therapist	Works with couples and families	Bachelor's degree, sometimes a master's degree, direct clinical training	American Association for Marriage and Family Therapy
Has good listening and communication skills	Psychiatrist	Must listen to patients and communicate treatments to them	Bachelor's degree, medical degree, certification exam	American Psychiatric Association
	Psychologist	Must listen to patients and communicate treatments to them	Doctoral degree, licensing exam	Society of Clinical Psychology, American Psychological Association
	Clinical social worker	Must listen to patients and communicate treatments to them	Master's degree, supervised clinical therapy	National Association of Social Workers
	Marriage and family therapist	Must listen to couples and families and communicate treatments to them	Bachelor's degree, sometimes a master's degree, direct clinical training	American Association for Marriage and Family Therapy
Enjoys working with families	Psychiatric nurse	Provides counseling to patients and their families	Nursing degree, specialized training in psychiatry and psychotherapy, direct clinical training	American Psychiatric Nurses Association
	Marriage and family therapist	Treats illnesses and disorders within families	Bachelor's degree, sometimes a master's degree, direct clinical training	American Association for Marriage and Family Therapy
Enjoys a variety of workplaces	Clinical social worker	May work in mental health clinics, schools, hospitals, or private practice	Master's degree, supervised clinical therapy	National Association of Social Workers
	Marriage and family therapist	May work in a social work setting or in private practice	Bachelor's degree, sometimes a master's degree, direct clinical training	American Association for Marriage and Family Therapy

(Continued)

Name _____

1. Which of these careers lines up best with your interests or personality?

_____

_____

_____

_____

_____

2. Choose one career to research further. For that career, visit the resource listed in the chart and compose a "day in the life" for someone with that career. Does this type of workday sound interesting to you?

_____

_____

_____

_____

_____

3. According to the chart, which level of education is necessary for your chosen career? Research community colleges and universities in your area and plot out an educational plan to follow if you want this career.

_____

_____

_____

_____

_____

4. Visit the *Occupational Outlook Handbook* online to research the job outlook for this particular career. Record your findings here.

_____

_____

_____

_____

_____

5. According to the *Occupational Outlook Handbook*, what is a typical salary for someone in this career?

_____

_____

_____

_____

_____

Chapter 17

Reading Practice

Reread the following passage from the textbook. Then answer the questions that follow.

Brain Injury

People who experience a serious brain injury are at greater risk of developing some mental illnesses and disorders. *Traumatic brain injury (TBI)* occurs when a severe blow or jolt to the head damages the brain. A *concussion* is a type of brain injury that results from a blow to the head or the body. Contact sports injuries and motor vehicle accidents are common causes of TBIs and concussions. Concussions result in disorientation, confusion, nausea, and weakness, and may cause memory loss or unconsciousness. Although usually temporary, concussions can lead to serious complications and should be treated by a doctor.

Brain injuries may cause temporary or permanent changes to brain function. Irreversible brain changes can result in depression, anxiety, personality changes, and aggression. People with brain injuries are also at greater risk of developing a substance abuse problem. In these situations, alcohol and drugs may be used in an attempt to regulate negative mood or pain.

_____ 1. What is the main idea of this passage?
  A. Contact sports injuries are dangerous.
  B. Concussions may result in loss of consciousness.
  C. People who experience brain injuries are at a greater risk of developing mental illnesses and disorders.
  D. Brain injuries may cause irreversible brain changes.

_____ 2. Which of the following describes a severe blow or jolt to the head that damages the brain?
  A. depression
  B. mental illness
  C. mental disorder
  D. traumatic brain injury

_____ 3. A(n) _____ is a type of brain injury that results from a blow to the head or the body..
  A. cranial distortion
  B. concussion
  C. schizophrenia
  D. arrhythmia

_____ 4. Which of the following is *not* a result of a concussion?
  A. disorientation
  B. tingling in the fingertips
  C. nausea
  D. weakness

Chapter 17

Practice Test

Completion: *Write the term that completes the statement in the space provided.*

1. People with _____ disorder have persistent and obsessive thoughts or feelings that they manage by engaging in ritualized behaviors.

2. _____ disorders are usually diagnosed in childhood and often cause problems with normal interpersonal interactions.

3. People with schizophrenia have higher-than-normal levels of the chemical _____ in their brains.

4. Traumatic life events can lead to _____ distortions in people's thinking.

5. People from certain family backgrounds may be at greater risk of attempting _____.

True/False: *Indicate whether each statement below is true or false by circling either T or F.*

T   F   6. The terms *mental illness* and *mental disorder* have different meanings.

T   F   7. Self-mutilation, or *cutting*, is the most common form of self-injury.

T   F   8. People with brain injuries are at a greater risk for developing a substance-abuse problem.

T   F   9. A pregnant woman's actions do not affect the mental health of her child.

T   F   10. People who experience long-term stress in their environments are more likely to attempt suicide.

Multiple Choice: *Write the letter that corresponds to the correct answer in the blank space.*

_____ 11. Extreme anxiety caused by specific objects or situations is called _____.
   A. disorder   C. phobia
   B. illness   D. stress

_____ 12. People with _____ anxiety disorder have a pattern of constantly worrying about many different activities and events.
   A. post-traumatic   C. depressive
   B. obsessive   D. generalized

_____ 13. Which of the following is *not* a typical symptom of major depression?
   A. sudden, manic moods   C. extreme tiredness and loss of energy
   B. difficulty concentrating   D. recurrent thoughts of death

_____ 14. The term *suicide* _____ describes a series of suicides in a community over a short period of time.
   A. *survivors*   C. *factors*
   B. *clusters*   D. *contagion*

_____ 15. _____ are used to make certain chemicals, such as serotonin, in the brain more available.
   A. Antidepressants   C. Lithium pills
   B. Control pills   D. Antipsychotics

Name _____ Date _____

Matching: *Match each key term to its definition by writing the letter of the term in the space provided.*

_____ 16. a medical condition in which a person experiences mental or emotional problems severe enough to interfere with daily functioning

_____ 17. the copying of suicide attempts after exposure to another person's suicide

_____ 18. people who lose a loved one to suicide

_____ 19. a negative or unfair belief circulated within society

_____ 20. a mental illness characterized by delusions, hallucinations, and irregular thought patterns

_____ 21. type of medication used to manage the symptoms of schizophrenia

_____ 22. hereditary vulnerabilities to various diseases and illnesses

A. antipsychotics

B. genetic predispositions

C. mental illness

D. schizophrenia

E. stigma

F. suicide contagion

G. survivors

Analyzing Data: *The graph below shows the percentage of teens 12 to 17 years of age who have experienced depressive symptoms, had suicidal thoughts, or attempted suicide. The data is organized by gender. Study the data in this graph and then answer the questions that follow.*

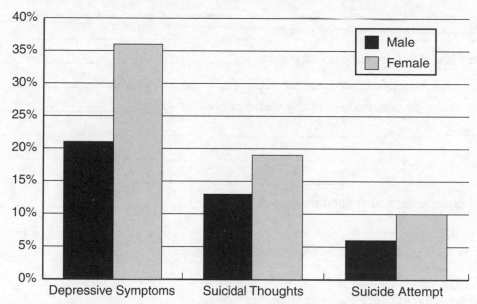

Depression and Suicide among Students 12–17 Years of Age

Source: The Office of Adolescent Health at the Department of Health and Human Services

23. What percent more females than males experienced depressive symptoms?

_____

24. What percent of males and females did *not* attempt suicide?

_____

Short Answer: *On a separate sheet of paper, answer the following questions using what you have learned in this chapter.*

25. What can you, as an individual, do to battle the social stigma surrounding mental illnesses and disorders?

26. What can you do to help a friend or family member who is suffering from a mental illness or disorder?

Lesson 18.1

Cultural Communication Differences

In chapter 18, you learned about the types of communication, but did you know that various cultures interpret verbal and nonverbal communication differently? For example, Americans often point with one finger to direct someone's attention to an object, but in some cultures, that is considered rude. Using reliable online sources, research four cultural communication differences and record your findings below. Be sure to determine whether the mode of communication is verbal or nonverbal, as well as the source of your information.

1. Explain the cultural communication difference: _____
   _____

   Is the communication difference primarily verbal or nonverbal? _____

   Online source: _____

   Describe a scenario in which the difference might occur: _____
   _____
   _____

2. Explain the cultural communication difference: _____
   _____

   Is the communication difference primarily verbal or nonverbal? _____

   Online source: _____
   _____
   _____

3. Explain the cultural communication difference: _____
   _____

   Is the communication difference primarily verbal or nonverbal? _____

   Online source: _____

   Describe a scenario in which the difference might occur: _____
   _____
   _____

4. Explain the cultural communication difference: _____
   _____

   Is the communication difference primarily verbal or nonverbal? _____

   Online source: _____

   Describe a scenario in which the difference might occur: _____
   _____
   _____

Lesson 18.1

Resolving Family Conflicts

Family relationships are some of the most important relationships you will have in your life; however, it's not uncommon for conflicts to arise between family members. The following scenarios describe conflicts between teenagers and members of their families. After reading each scenario, offer each teen your advice for resolving the conflict.

1. Drew and his younger brother, Michael, are only a year apart. Last month, Michael got his driver's license and now he wants to use the car all the time. The two brothers are constantly fighting over who gets to drive the car. Since he's the oldest, Drew thinks he should be able to use the car more often than Michael. Their parents are sick of the fighting and have threatened to take the car away from both of them. What advice would you give Drew and Michael about resolving their conflict?

   _____

   _____

   _____

   _____

2. Isaac is pushing his parents to give him a later curfew. He has to be home by 10:00 p.m. on weekends, but all of his friends stay out until 10:30. Isaac doesn't understand why his parents won't extend his curfew—especially since it's only by a half hour. Every weekend night he goes out, he feels angry with his parents. What advice would you give Isaac and his parents about resolving their conflict?

   _____

   _____

   _____

   _____

3. Rafael's parents always tell him to put his cell phone away at the dinner table. Rafael can't understand why they get so upset—it doesn't take him long to send a text message or two between bites. It seems like he's always fighting with his parents about how much time he spends on his phone. Sometimes his parents even take his phone away. What advice would you give Rafael and his parents about resolving their conflict?

   _____

   _____

   _____

   _____

4. Olivia's younger sister, Chloe, has been getting on her nerves lately. Chloe comes into Olivia's room without knocking and she keeps wearing Olivia's clothes without asking. Yesterday, Olivia wanted to wear her favorite sweater, but she couldn't because Chloe had worn it and spilled spaghetti sauce all down the front. What advice would you give Olivia and Chloe about resolving their conflict?

   _____

   _____

   _____

   _____

Lesson 18.2

Giving Friendship Advice

Making new friends can be a challenge, especially if you are new to an environment or community. Imagine you are the first person to welcome Jessica, a new student at your school. What advice would you give her about making new friends? For this activity, share six strategies that you learned in your textbook or that have worked well for you in the past. Then, share six strategies for developing healthy friendships and being a good friend. Compare your responses with a classmate.

Strategies for making new friends:

1. _____
   _____

2. _____
   _____

3. _____
   _____

4. _____
   _____

5. _____
   _____

6. _____
   _____

Strategies for developing healthy friendships:

1. _____
   _____

2. _____
   _____

3. _____
   _____

4. _____
   _____

5. _____
   _____

6. _____
   _____

Lesson 18.3

Healthy versus Unhealthy Dating Relationships

Many people experience their first dating relationships during their teenage years. Learning how to distinguish between healthy and unhealthy dating relationships is an important skill. Read the following stories about teenagers and their dating relationships. Decide whether each couple seems to have a healthy or unhealthy dating relationship, and then explain how you came to that conclusion.

1. Chris and Hannah have been dating for three months. Hannah really likes Chris, but he's been acting jealous lately. Every day, he asks whom she is texting and gets upset if it's one of her male friends. Last week Hannah's friend Blake gave her a ride to the football game, and Chris was so angry he wouldn't speak to her for the rest of the night.

   A. Is this dating relationship healthy or unhealthy? _____

   B. Why? _____

   _____

   _____

2. Kai and Andy are involved in a lot of extracurricular activities, but they try to support each other as much as they can. Kai attends as many of Andy's baseball games as her busy rehearsal schedule allows; and when Kai was the lead in the school play, no one cheered louder for her than Andy.

   A. Is this dating relationship healthy or unhealthy? _____

   B. Why? _____

   _____

   _____

3. When Easton and Abby started dating last May, they had an open, honest discussion about how much time they should spend together. While they enjoy each other's friends, they decided that they should both make time to hang out with their friends alone. Last Friday, Easton went to a hockey game with his friends, while Abby had two of her friends over to watch a movie. On Saturday, the couple went out for ice cream together.

   A. Is this dating relationship healthy or unhealthy? _____

   B. Why? _____

   _____

4. Each morning, Owen leaves the house early so he can pick up his girlfriend, Katie, on his way to school. He tries to give Katie thoughtful gifts and do nice things for her, such as offering her rides because she doesn't have a car. Lately, though, Owen has been feeling like he's just Katie's chauffeur. When she forgot his birthday last week, his feelings were really hurt.

   A. Is this dating relationship healthy or unhealthy? _____

   B. Why? _____

   _____

   _____

Chapter 18

Reading Practice

Reread the following passage from the textbook. Then answer the questions that follow.

Verbal Communication

Verbal communication involves the use of words to send an oral (spoken) or written message. You use verbal communication all the time—through everyday conversation, text messages, phone calls, e-mails, social media posts, letters, and notes. For example, telling a parent you will be home at a certain time is a form of verbal communication.

Nonverbal Communication

Communication involves more than just words. You also communicate with your face and body. ***Nonverbal communication*** involves communicating through facial expressions, body language, gestures, tone and volume of voice, and other signals that do not involve the use of words. Your nonverbal communication shows people whether or not you are paying attention and are interested in the conversation. These signals are an especially important part of showing respect for the person communicating with you.

Nonverbal communication includes

* eye contact or lack of eye contact;
* facial expressions, such as smiling, frowning, or eye rolling;
* gestures, such as nodding, shaking the head, or moving the hands;
* posture, such as learning forward, facing away, or slumping in a chair;
* tone of voice, such as friendliness, doubt, or sarcasm;
* volume of voice, such as loud or soft; and
* *intonation*, or pitch of voice, such as high-pitched or low-pitched.

_____ 1. Text messages, phone calls, e-mails, and social media posts are examples of _____.
   A. verbal communication
   B. nonverbal communication
   C. both verbal and nonverbal communication
   D. none of the above

_____ 2. Facial expressions, gestures, and voice tone and volume are examples of _____.
   A. verbal communication
   B. nonverbal communication
   C. both verbal and nonverbal communication
   D. none of the above

_____ 3. Nonverbal communication shows others whether or not you _____.
   A. are showing respect
   B. are paying attention
   C. are interested in the conversation
   D. all of the above

Chapter 18

Practice Test

Completion: *Write the term that completes the statement in the space provided.*

1. Eye contact is a form of _____ communication.

2. Competing with siblings for various material or nonmaterial items is called

   _____.

3. A(n) _____ is a small group of friends who deliberately exclude other people from joining.

4. Attraction without closeness is called a(n) _____.

5. Feelings of _____ are based largely on physical attraction.

True/False: *Indicate whether each statement below is true or false by circling either T or F.*

T   F   6. Good communication requires good listening skills.

T   F   7. Relationships that are full of tension and conflict can negatively affect your health.

T   F   8. Peer pressure can be both positive and negative.

T   F   9. Being a good friend means expressing your feelings openly during conflicts.

T   F   10. Your individuality becomes less important when you enter a dating relationship.

Multiple Choice: *Write the letter that corresponds to the correct answer in the blank space.*

_____ 11. Which of the following is a sign of an unhealthy relationship?
- A. You have been physically assaulted by your partner.
- B. You feel you cannot say anything right.
- C. You are made fun of.
- D. all of the above

_____ 12. Which of the following is true of family relationships?
- A. They provide for physical needs.
- B. They serve to educate and socialize children.
- C. They meet mental and emotional needs.
- D. all of the above

_____ 13. Strategies for maintaining healthy relationships with your parents or caregivers include _____.
- A. not discussing family rules
- B. following your family's rules, even if you disagree with them
- C. keeping information your family wouldn't like to know a secret
- D. avoiding spending time together if you are not getting along

_____ 14. Diversity is present in a group of people with various backgrounds, including different _____.
- A. ages
- B. ethnicities
- C. genders
- D. all of the above

_____ 15. Which of the following is a strategy for forming a healthy dating relationship?
- A. finding ways to cope with your nerves
- B. avoiding group dating
- C. entering into a new relationship as soon as a previous relationship ends
- D. spending your free time exclusively with your new boyfriend or girlfriend

Name _____ Date _____

Matching: *Match each term to its definition by writing the letter of the term in the space provided.*

_____ 16. a small group of friends who intentionally turn away people who may want to interact with or befriend them

_____ 17. being romantically involved with only one partner

_____ 18. individuals with whom you interact regularly but may not consider to be friends

_____ 19. competitive feelings and behaviors that exist between siblings

_____ 20. the practice of concentrating on what a person is saying

_____ 21. the act of forcing someone into sexual activity that he or she does not want

_____ 22. a response that signals a message has been received and understood

A. sexual assault

B. clique

C. acquaintances

D. sibling rivalry

E. feedback

F. exclusive

G. active listening

Analyzing Data: *Use the information provided to answer the following questions. Assume that 1,500 teenagers were included in this survey.*

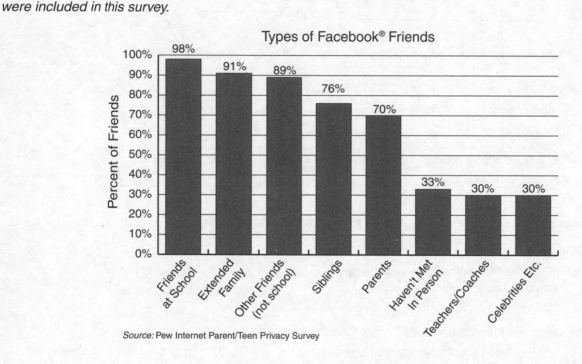

Types of Facebook® Friends

Source: Pew Internet Parent/Teen Privacy Survey

23. How many teenagers are Facebook® friends with someone they haven't met in person?

_____

24. Analyze your social media friendships. About what percentage of your Facebook® friends are from each of these groups?

_____

Short Answer: *On a separate sheet of paper, answer the following questions using what you have learned in this chapter.*

25. What are five important qualities of healthy dating relationships?

26. What are three common problems in friendships?

Key Terms Review

Multiple Choice: *Write the letter that corresponds to the correct answer in the blank space.*

_____ 1. _____ is a settlement of a disagreement in which each side gives in a little to the other.
A. Arbitration
B. Mediation
C. Compromise
D. Capitulation

_____ 2. A(n) _____ is a neutral third party who helps resolve conflicts by listening carefully to each perspective.
A. auditor
B. mediator
C. judge
D. aggressor

_____ 3. People who are _____ speak honestly about and act appropriately in response to their feelings, needs, and goals.
A. assertive
B. aggressive
C. antagonistic
D. peacemakers

_____ 4. _____ is a method of resolving conflict in which a neutral peer listens to both parties in a disagreement and helps them achieve a solution.
A. Adjudication
B. Peer counseling
C. Peer investigation
D. Peer mediation

_____ 5. A person who exhibits this type of behavior speaks or acts in a demanding and insulting way.
A. passive
B. aggressive
C. assertive
D. passive-aggressive

_____ 6. _____ is the threat or use of physical force to injure another person.
A. Intimidation
B. Listening
C. Mediation
D. Assault

_____ 7. _____ is a type of aggressive behavior in which someone intentionally and repeatedly causes another person injury or discomfort.
A. Bullying
B. Assertiveness
C. Aggressiveness
D. Hazing

(Continued)

_____ 8. _____ is violent behavior that occurs on school property or at school events.
   A. Institutional violence
   B. School violence
   C. Community violence
   D. Educational violence

_____ 9. _____ is any humiliating or dangerous activity that someone is required to perform, often to be accepted by a group.
   A. Aggression
   B. Bullying
   C. Assault
   D. Hazing

Matching: *Match each definition to its corresponding term by writing the letter of the term in the blank space.*

_____ 10. a synonym for *murder*

_____ 11. the act of looking at, or ogling, someone for sexual pleasure

_____ 12. failure to meet the basic physical, emotional, medical, or educational needs of someone dependent upon others to fulfill these needs; also, failure to provide protection from harm as a result of inadequate supervision or exposure to a dangerous living situation

_____ 13. any abuse or neglect that harms or seeks to harm a child

_____ 14. any abuse or neglect that harms or seeks to harm an older adult

_____ 15. a form of abuse that involves using a child for sexual stimulation

A. child abuse

B. child sexual abuse

C. elder abuse

D. homicide

E. neglect

F. voyeurism

Defining Terms: *Write the definition of each term in the blank space.*

16. *consent:* _____

_____

17. *domestic violence:* _____

_____

18. *sexual harassment:* _____

_____

19. *rape:* _____

_____

20. *sexual violence:* _____

_____

21. *acquaintance rape:* _____

_____

22. *statutory rape:* _____

_____

Lesson 19.1

Resolving Conflict

Conflict is a normal part of everyday life, and it is not always bad. Engaging in conflict can have positive outcomes for yourself and your relationships. Understanding conflict—including what causes conflict and how best to prevent and resolve conflict—is important in developing and maintaining healthy relationships with others. For each scenario described below, explain how a resolution might be achieved.

1. Vincent's friend Jamey is having a party at his house on Saturday. Vincent knows, however, that his parents think Jamey is a negative influence and will not let him go. Jamey drinks alcohol, smokes marijuana, and occasionally skips classes at school. When Vincent approaches his parents about attending the party, they tell him that they will not discuss the matter and that they don't want Vincent to interact with Jamey outside of school. Vincent gets angry, leaves the room, and goes to his bedroom, slamming the door. What can Vincent and his parents do to resolve this conflict?

   _____

   _____

   _____

2. Mariska and George have been dating for a year. Mariska is involved in several extracurricular organizations and activities, and she finds it hard to spend quality time with George as well as her friends amid her hectic schedule. One afternoon, George tells Mariska that he is not happy with the way their relationship has been going. He irritably delivers an ultimatum: "You will reevaluate your priorities, or I will break up with you." What can George and Mariska do to resolve this conflict?

   _____

   _____

   _____

3. Steve and Jack are in the same trigonometry class. While Jack is doing exceptionally well in trigonometry, Steve is exasperated because he has been struggling to understand the material. Because Steve sits next to Jack in class, he asks Jack to let him copy his answers to the test questions. Jack replies, "Are you serious? I'm not jeopardizing my college scholarship so you can cheat, loser." Steve angrily tells his friend, "Thanks a lot. I'd help you out if you needed it." He gathers his books before issuing a sullen good-bye and leaves. What could Steve and Jack have done to resolve this conflict?

   _____

   _____

   _____

4. Marguerite's parents have asked her to babysit her 12-year-old sister on Saturday night so they can go out for a movie and dinner. Because of their busy work schedules, Marguerite's parents have not gone on a "date" or otherwise spent much time together for the past five months. Marguerite explains that the boy she likes at school has finally asked her for a date—on Saturday night. She is concerned that if she cancels the date, she will not be asked out again. "I always get stuck babysitting," Marguerite complains. What can Marguerite and her parents do to resolve this conflict?

   _____

   _____

   _____

Lessons 19.2

What Would You Do?

For each scenario described below, briefly state what you would do to help manage or prevent the abuse from escalating. Then, find a partner, and share what you would do. Record your partner's answers beside yours and discuss the differences in your responses.

1. One of your friends has become a victim of cyberbullying. Other students at school have been taunting and threatening her on social media sites, and she has grown increasingly distressed and despondent. She explains that her parents have talked to the school principal, but to no avail. What would you do in this situation?

   _____

   _____

   _____

   What would your partner do?_____

   _____

   _____

   _____

2. A new student who is a Muslim has begun to attend your school. Almost immediately, she starts to receive anonymous, threatening letters; and other students routinely make insulting remarks about her religion, clothing, and ethnicity. One afternoon, you witness someone pushing her and tossing her books onto the floor. What would you do in this situation?

   _____

   _____

   _____

   What would your partner do?_____

   _____

   _____

   _____

3. One day, while standing at your school locker, you observe a classmate being violently slapped in the face by his girlfriend. The girl is shrieking at the boy, who reels back, stunned. What would you do in this situation?

   _____

   _____

   _____

   What would your partner do?_____

   _____

   _____

   _____

Name _____

4. A classmate frequently comes to school with bruises and lacerations on his skin. On one occasion, he arrives to class with a black eye. He keeps to himself, is painfully shy, and avoids eye contact. What would you do in this situation?

_____

_____

_____

What would your partner do?_____

_____

_____

5. You learn through the grapevine at school that two of the boys in your class are plotting to "exact revenge" on those who have bullied them. You hear that the boys are planning to bring weapons to school. What would you do in this situation?

_____

_____

_____

What would your partner do?_____

_____

_____

6. A young boy in your neighborhood is always outside, unsupervised, regardless of weather conditions. He is clearly underweight, and his clothes are tattered and too small for him. He does not appear to have any bruises, and he doesn't exhibit any other obvious signs of abuse. What would you do in this situation?

_____

_____

_____

What would your partner do?_____

_____

_____

Lesson 19.4

Taking Precautions

Teenagers are especially vulnerable to unwanted sexual activity, sexual abuse, and date rape. It is important to remember that being a victim of sexual assault is never your fault. You should, however, do everything in your power to ensure your personal safety. Read each of the scenarios presented below and identify what each person should do to ensure his or her safety and avoid becoming a victim of sexual assault. Refer to the Skills for Health and Wellness feature on page 579 of your textbook if you need help.

1. Bianca is at a party that a few of her friends are throwing for graduation. She is talking to a boy named Steve, who is very charming and interesting. So far, it seems that Steve and Bianca share a lot of interests and hobbies. Bianca is enjoying herself until Steve suddenly says that he has to show her something in the kitchen. Bianca thinks this is strange, and it seems even stranger when Steve insists that she put down her drink so he can take her hand and lead her into the kitchen. What should Bianca do?

   _____

   _____

   _____

   _____

   _____

2. Damien and Rosalie are studying for an exam in their health class. They are at Rosalie's house, and her parents are out for the evening. Before Damien and Rosalie have finished their practice test, Rosalie suggests that they take some pictures. She removes her smartphone from her backpack, turns on the camera, and tells Damien to remove his clothes. "No," he replies, "I don't want any pictures of myself like that floating in cyberspace." Rosalie is insistent. Damien is worried she won't take no for an answer. What should Damien do?

   _____

   _____

   _____

   _____

   _____

3. Ellie is hanging out with some friends and with the boy she has a crush on, Jacob. Everyone is getting along well and having a good time. Ellie and Jacob spend a long time chatting with each other. As it gets late, several people begin to arrange carpools to get back home. Jacob offers to drive Ellie home. Ellie appreciates the offer, but she doesn't know Jacob very well. Although she has had a crush on him for a while, tonight is the first time she's gotten to talk to him properly. What should Ellie do?

   _____

   _____

   _____

   _____

   _____

4. Thursday night, while he's working on an essay for class, Matthias gets a text message from one of his friends. There's a big party going on the next night and Matthias is invited. Matthias' friend tells him that no adults will be at the party, so it will be extra fun. Matthias's friend also tells him that there will probably be alcohol at the party, so it's best if he doesn't tell his parents where he is going. What should Matthias do?

_____

_____

_____

_____

_____

5. Chantel and a few of her friends have an important chemistry test coming up. They all meet at the public library after school to study and are there all afternoon and evening. Chantel's friends are picked up by their parents, but Chantel borrowed the family's minivan to drive herself home. Everyone leaves the library when it closes at 9:00 p.m., and Chantel must walk to her car alone in the dark parking lot. What should Chantel do?

_____

_____

_____

_____

_____

6. Winnie and her little brother, David, have part-time jobs working at a local grocery store. One evening, they both work the late shift and have to close the store. No one is able to pick them up this late, so they have to walk home late at night through a bad part of town. Though they are nervous, Winnie and David try to be aware of their surroundings at all times. They notice a car driving up next to them and slowing down. A man inside the car asks if they would like a ride. He seems like a clean-cut young man, and Winnie and David are tired after their long shifts at work. What should Winnie and David do?

_____

_____

_____

_____

Lesson 19.4

The Importance of Consent

Consent is a direct, verbal agreement that occurs when someone clearly says yes. Consent does not occur if someone says no *or does* not *say anything at all. Under certain situations, some people are not legally capable of giving consent. Review the section on consent in your textbook. Then read the following scenarios to determine whether consent has been given in each. Explain each answer.*

1. Fifteen-year-old Jenny is excited to be at a party thrown by a group of college students. A college student named Brad approaches Jenny, and she is surprised that he wants to talk to her. Brad asks if she wants to have sex. Jenny agrees. Has consent been given? Why or why not?

   _____

   _____

   _____

   _____

   _____

2. Ben, who is 26 years old, is at a party. By the time guests begin to leave, Ben is so intoxicated that he can barely stand up. On the way upstairs, Ben tells his friend Cassie that he likes her dress. Cassie is surprised because she always liked Ben but assumed he didn't like her. She asks him if he'd like to have sex, and he mumbles an agreement. Has consent been given? Why or why not?

   _____

   _____

   _____

   _____

   _____

3. After a party, 22-year-old Brianna is left alone with her boyfriend, Jake. Jake asks if she wants to have sex. Brianna knows that she doesn't want to have sex, but when she tells Jake, Jake makes fun of her, calling her a "prude." Feeling pressured and embarrassed, Brianna gives in. Has consent been given? Why or why not?

   _____

   _____

   _____

   _____

   _____

   _____

Chapter 19

Reading Practice

Reread the following passage from the textbook. Then answer the questions that follow.

Consequences of Child Abuse

Your sense of well-being comes from knowing that you have the love, support, and respect of your family members and caregivers. When people are abused or neglected, their sense of well-being is shattered. Not surprisingly, that can have serious consequences. People who experience abuse may also suffer physical injuries.

A child who is abused may experience short- and long-term physical and psychological problems. Each year an estimated 750,000 children and teenagers—or 85 children *every single hour*—are treated for abuse-related injuries in hospital emergency departments in the United States. Almost 2,000 children in the United States die from abuse or neglect each year.

Physical consequences of abuse may include brain damage, blindness, motor impairments, and cognitive impairments. Abused children are also more likely than others to develop health problems and diseases as adults, including heart disease, cancer, liver disease, and obesity.

Children who are abused are also more likely than others to behave in ways that can harm their health. Abused children have an increased risk of

- smoking;
- becoming alcoholics;
- abusing drugs;
- engaging in high-risk sexual behaviors;
- being delinquent;
- doing poorly in school and failing to graduate from high school; and
- being arrested as juveniles and adults.

Not surprisingly, children who are abused or neglected are also at greater risk of experiencing psychological problems. The psychological problems experienced by abused or neglected children include depression, anxiety, eating disorders, and post-traumatic stress disorder. The stress of ongoing, or chronic, abuse may also cause children to develop learning, attention, and memory problems. These problems increase the likelihood that abused children will struggle in school.

Finally, child abuse can impair a person's ability to establish and maintain healthy intimate relationships in adulthood. People who do not experience love, trust, and support in their early relationships may have trouble building healthy relationships with others later.

Fortunately, children who have been abused are not doomed to an unhappy and unhealthy life. They can get help to feel better about themselves and others, and live fulfilling lives.

_____ 1. Which statement best expresses the main idea of this passage?

    A. A child who is abused may experience short- and long-term physical and psychological problems.

    B. The stress of ongoing, or chronic, abuse may cause children to develop learning, attention, and memory problems.

    C. Abused children have an increased risk of substance abuse.

    D. People who suffer child abuse may have trouble building healthy relationships with others later.

(Continued)

_____ 2. Approximately how many children and teenagers in the United States are treated each year for abuse-related injuries in hospital emergency departments?

    A. 85

    B. 2,000

    C. 750,000

    D. 950,000

_____ 3. Abused children are at increased risk for developing which of the following habits?

    A. abusing alcohol

    B. abusing drugs

    C. smoking

    D. all of the above

_____ 4. Which of the following statements is *not* true of children who have been abused or neglected?

    A. They often experience psychological problems such as depression, anxiety, eating disorders, and post-traumatic stress disorder.

    B. They can have difficulty establishing and maintaining healthy, intimate relationships in adulthood.

    C. The stress of chronic abuse or neglect may cause them to develop learning, attention, and memory problems.

    D. none of the above

_____ 5. Which of the following statements best explains the importance of love, trust, and support in one's early relationships?

    A. People who do not experience love, trust, and support in their early relationships may have trouble building healthy relationships with others in adulthood.

    B. Victims of child abuse are less likely to desire love, trust, and support from other people in adulthood.

    C. People who have suffered child abuse or neglect tend to experience more intense relationships as adults.

    D. There is no correlation between child abuse and the ability to cultivate healthy relationships later in life.

Chapter 19

Practice Test

Completion: *Write the term that completes the statement in the space provided.*

1. _____ is a method of resolving conflict in which a neutral peer listens to both parties in a disagreement and helps them achieve a solution.

2. A _____ involves each side of a disagreement giving in a little to each other.

3. People who are _____ speak honestly about and act appropriately in response to their feelings, needs, and goals.

4. A _____ is a neutral third party who helps parties achieve conflict resolution.

5. Unlike assertive behavior, which is a healthy form of expression, _____ behavior is insulting and demanding.

True/False: *Indicate whether each statement below is true or false by circling either T or F.*

T   F   6. Assault is a physical action; it does not include threatening behavior.

T   F   7. Each year in the United States, approximately one out of every seven children between 2 and 17 years of age experiences some form of abuse or neglect.

T   F   8. Child neglect occurs when a child's basic physical, emotional, medical, or educational needs are not met by his or her parents or guardians.

T   F   9. Voyeurism is *not* a form of child sexual abuse.

T   F   10. Elder abuse is typically committed by family members or paid caregivers.

T   F   11. Bullying is a form of aggressive behavior that is intentional but is not usually repeated.

T   F   12. Domestic violence occurs only between married couples.

T   F   13. Hazing is any humiliating or dangerous activity that someone is required to perform, often as part of being accepted by a group.

T   F   14. The definition of *school violence* includes any violent behavior that occurs on school property, on school buses, or at school-sponsored events.

T   F   15. Sometimes sexual assault or abuse can be the fault of the victim.

T   F   16. Consent is when someone doesn't say no to sexual activity.

Matching: *Match each key term to its definition by writing the letter of the term in the space provided.*

_____ 17. any form of sexual activity that is attempted without the other person's consent

_____ 18. a form of sexual violence that involves nonconsensual sexual intercourse

_____ 19. sexual activity that occurs between an adult and an adolescent

_____ 20. any form of unwanted sexual attention

_____ 21. unwanted sexual intercourse that is committed by someone the victim knows

_____ 22. a direct, verbal, noncoerced agreement from someone who is capable of making an informed decision

A.   acquaintance rape

B.   consent

C.   rape

D.   sexual harassment

E.   sexual violence

F.   statutory rape

(Continued)

Name _____

Short Answer: *Even highly-trained experts cannot predict with certainty whether a person will engage in violence. However, behavioral experts do know that the confluence of certain psychological and environmental factors can make a person more likely to engage in violence. Briefly describe how each of the factors listed below affects a person's likelihood to engage in violence.*

23. Mental or emotional state

_____

_____

_____

_____

_____

24. Exposure to violence

_____

_____

_____

_____

_____

25. Alcohol and/or drug use

_____

_____

_____

_____

_____

26. Personal gain

_____

_____

_____

_____

_____

27. Availability of a weapon

_____

_____

_____

_____

_____

Lesson 20.1

Key Terms Review

Multiple Choice: *Write the letter that corresponds to the correct answer in the blank space.*

_____ 1. A(n) _____ is the male sex cell, which combines with the female sex cell to create a zygote.

    A. semen   C. ovum

    B. sperm   D. gamete

_____ 2. What is the name of the female sex cell?

    A. semen   C. ovum

    B. sperm   D. gamete

_____ 3. Cells increase in a number through a process called _____.

    A. sexual reproduction   C. asexual reproduction

    B. cell division   D. fertilization

_____ 4. The term *zygote* describes which of the following?

    A. an ovum before it is fertilized by a   C. an ovum that has been fertilized by a
          sperm   sperm

    B. an ovum that was not fertilized   D. none of the above

_____ 5. In sexual reproduction, each parent contributes a sex cell, called a _____.

    A. gamete   C. chromosome

    B. zygote   D. embryo

_____ 6. The male and female sex cells combine during the process of _____.

    A. mitosis   C. fertilization

    B. asexual reproduction   D. meiosis

Matching: *Match each term to its definition by writing the letter of the term in the space provided.*

_____ 7. a type of gene that is always expressed in offspring

_____ 8. a type of cell division in which a cell splits its own genetic material and then divides into two different cells

_____ 9. the process by which the genetic material of two organisms—one male and one female—combine to create offspring

_____ 10. a process that requires only one cell and which produces offspring identical to that cell

_____ 11. a type of cell division in which a cell copies its own genetic material and then divides into two identical cells

_____ 12. a type of gene that is not always expressed in offspring

    A. dominant

    B. recessive

    C. sexual reproduction

    D. asexual reproduction

    E. mitosis

    F. meiosis

Lesson 20.1

Dominant and Recessive Traits

Some genes are dominant, and others are recessive. If you receive a dominant gene from either parent, you will exhibit the dominant trait. Recessive traits are only exhibited if you receive recessive genes from each parent. The table below identifies physical characteristics as dominant or recessive. Using this table, assess your own physical characteristics and, if possible, compare your traits to your parents' traits. In the left column, check which traits you possess. Then, in the columns labeled Mother *and* Father, *write* R *(for* recessive*) or* D *(for* dominant*) depending on which traits your parents possess. Answer the questions that follow.*

Trait D—dominant R—recessive	Mother	Father
___ Widow's peak (D) ___ Straight hairline (R)		
___ Brown eye color (D) ___ Nonbrown eye color (R)		
___ Cleft in chin (D) ___ No cleft in chin (R)		
___ Freckles (D) ___ No freckles (R)		
___ Able to roll tongue (D) ___ Unable to roll tongue (R)		
___ Earlobes hang free from head (D) ___ Earlobes attached to head (R)		
___ Little finger bends inward at last joint (D) ___ Little finger is straight (R)		
___ Cheek dimples (D) ___ No dimples (R)		

1. Do you have more dominant traits or recessive traits?

_____

2. Were you surprised by any of the traits you or your parents possessed? Why or why not?

_____

_____

Lesson 20.2

The Female Reproductive System

Label the figure below with the appropriate terms from the list provided.

Terms

body of uterus	ovaries
cervical canal	ovum
cervix	ureter
endometrium	uterine blood vessels
fallopian tubes	uterus cavity
ovarian blood vessels	vagina

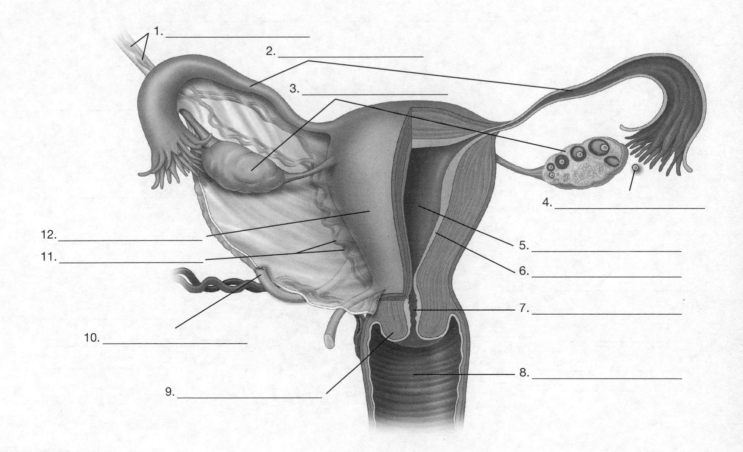

1. _____

2. _____

3. _____

4. _____

5. _____

6. _____

7. _____

8. _____

9. _____

10. _____

11. _____

12. _____

Body Scientific International, LLC

Lesson 20.2

The Male Reproductive System

Label the figure below with the appropriate terms from the list provided.

Terms

anus	scrotum
epididymis	seminal vesicle
external urethral orifice	testis
foreskin	ureter
glans penis	urethra
penis	urinary bladder
prostate	vas deferens
rectum	

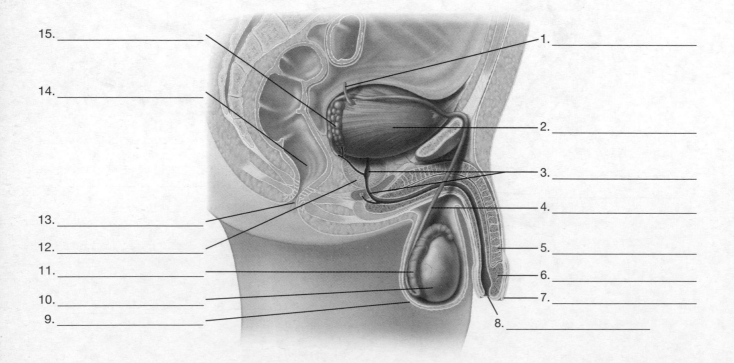

15. _____

14. _____

13. _____

12. _____

11. _____

10. _____

9. _____

1. _____

2. _____

3. _____

4. _____

5. _____

6. _____

7. _____

8. _____

Lesson 20.3

Key Terms Review

Multiple Choice: *Write the letter that corresponds to the correct answer in the blank space.*

_____ 1. During pregnancy, a woman should make regular visits to her _____.
   A. podiatrist
   B. obstetrician/gynecologist (OB/GYN)
   C. dermatologist
   D. ophthalmologist

_____ 2. _____ is the hormone that signals pregnancy.
   A. Insulin
   B. Chorionic gonadotropin
   C. Glucose
   D. Thyroxine

_____ 3. The process by which embryonic cells develop into cells with specific structures and functions is called _____.
   A. differentiation
   B. organogenesis
   C. cleavage
   D. implantation

_____ 4. The _____ is the membrane that develops around the implanted embryo.
   A. amnion
   B. placenta
   C. chorion
   D. blastocyst

_____ 5. The process by which a single-celled zygote divides into many cells is known as which of the following?
   A. implantation
   B. differentiation
   C. fertilization
   D. cleavage

_____ 6. Which of the following structures connects the developing fetus to the placenta?
   A. uterus
   B. amnion
   C. umbilical cord
   D. embryo

_____ 7. Organs belonging to the developing fetus take their familiar locations in the body during _____.
   A. cleavage
   B. differentiation
   C. organocytosis
   D. organogenesis

Matching: *Match each term to its definition by writing the letter of the term in the space provided.*

_____ 8. embryonic tissues that will eventually constitute the three main types of tissues in the body

_____ 9. a ball of cells formed by the cleaving zygote, and which implants in the uterus

_____ 10. a membrane that forms a fluid-filled sac, which cushions and protects a developing fetus

_____ 11. the merged chorion and endometrial tissue that surrounds, protects, and nurtures a developing fetus

_____ 12. the period of time between fertilization of an ovum and the birth of a baby

A. amnion

B. gestation

C. germ layers

D. blastocyst

E. placenta

Lesson 20.3

Cleavage and Implantation

Label the figure below with the appropriate terms from the list provided.

Terms

2 days	myometrium
3 days	ovary
4 days	ovum
7 days (blastocyst)	sperm
cavity of uterus	uterine/fallopian tube
endometrium	uterus
fertilization	zygote (fertilized egg)

1. _____   3. _____   5. _____

2. _____   4. _____

14. _____

13. _____

12. _____

11. _____

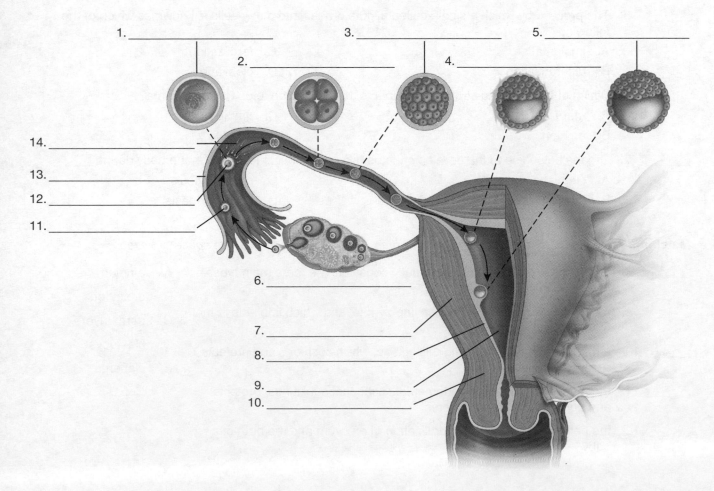

6. _____

7. _____

8. _____

9. _____

10. _____

Lesson 20.4

Create a Pregnancy Care Plan

Melanie and her husband, Brad, are expecting their first child in the spring. Unlike you, Melanie never took a health course in high school, and therefore does not know what to expect for her pregnancy. For this activity, create a pregnancy care plan for Melanie by filling in the information below.

Doctor's Appointments

1. Recommended frequency: _____

   _____

2. What to expect at the first appointment: _____

   _____

   _____

   _____

3. What to expect at follow-up appointments: _____

   _____

   _____

   _____

Food and Nutrition

4. Normal amount of weight gain: _____

5. Number of calories to add to daily diet: _____

6. Foods and substances to avoid: _____

   _____

   _____

   _____

   _____

Physical Activity

7. Physical activity recommendations: _____

   _____

   _____

   _____

   _____

   _____

   _____

Lesson 20.5

Key Terms Review

Multiple Choice: *Write the letter that corresponds to the correct answer in the blank space.*

_____ 1. The ability to produce children is known as _____.
    A. epididymitis   C. premenstrual syndrome
    B. endometriosis   D. fertility

_____ 2. The symptoms of _____ start one to two weeks before menstruation and cause cramps, bloating, and mood changes.
    A. premenstrual syndrome (PMS)   C. ovarian cysts
    B. endometriosis   D. none of the above

_____ 3. _____ is the inflammation of the testes, which leads to pain, swelling, and possible penile discharge.
    A. Testicular cancer   C. Cryptorchidism
    B. Prostate cancer   D. Orchitis

_____ 4. The inflammation of the epididymus is known as _____.
    A. epididymitis   C. cryptorchidism
    B. prostatitis   D. prostate cancer

_____ 5. Which of the following is the second most common cancer in the world?
    A. testicular cancer   C. uterine cancer
    B. prostate cancer   D. ovarian cancer

_____ 6. _____ is a condition in which the symptoms of PMS become severe enough to interfere with a woman's day-to-day life.
    A. Extreme premenstrual syndrome (PMS)   C. Endometriosis
    B. Premenstrual dysphoric disorder (PMDD)   D. Uterine cancer

Matching: *Match each term to its definition by writing the letter of the term in the space provided.*

_____ 7. a benign tumor that grows in the uterine muscle   A. uterine cancer

_____ 8. a type of cancer that grows in the endometrium   B. ovarian cancer

_____ 9. a condition in which the testes fail to descend from the abdominal cavity   C. ovarian cysts

                                                                   D. cryptorchidism

_____ 10. a type of cancer that grows in the ovaries   E. fibroid

_____ 11. a type of cancer that grows in one or both of the testes   F. testicular cancer

_____ 12. noncancerous tumors on the ovaries

Lesson 20.5

Diseases and Disorders of the Reproductive System

Both the male and female reproductive systems can be vulnerable to a variety of diseases and disorders. Using the information you learned in this chapter, fill in the missing information in the table below.

Disease/Disorder	Male or Female	Definition	Symptoms	Treatments
Endometriosis				
Prostatitis				
Ovarian cysts				
Epididymitis				
Orchitis				
Testicular cancer				
Premenstrual syndrome (PMS)				

Chapter 20

Reading Practice

Reread the following passage from the textbook. Then answer the questions that follow.

Male Cancers

Adolescent males should be aware of a few cancers that can affect their reproductive organs. The sooner these cancers are detected, the easier they are to treat.

Testicular Cancer

Testicular cancer is cancer that is present in one or both testes. Men who experience testicular swelling or feel a painless lump on a testicle should see their physician. Men may also experience aching in the lower abdomen or scrotum as a symptom. A testicular examination should be part of a general physical examination, and young men should conduct regular self-exams.

The cause of testicular cancer is unknown, but known risk factors include cryptorchidism and a family history of testicular cancer. Fortunately, early testicular cancer is treatable.

Prostate Cancer

The signs and symptoms of *prostate cancer* resemble those of prostatitis. A male's age is the single most important risk factor for prostate cancer—most cases occur in men who are 65 years of age or older. Other risk factors include smoking, a high-fat diet, and prostatitis.

Screening tests for prostate cancer exist, but men should consult their doctor about whether they need to have the tests. They are usually given annually after a man reaches 40 years of age. Prostate screening involves the *prostate-specific antigen (PSA)* test, which measures the amount of a substance produced by the prostate that is present in the blood. A doctor also performs a digital rectal exam by inserting fingers (digits) inside the rectum, where the surface of the prostate can be felt.

_____ 1. Symptoms of testicular cancer include _____.
   A. aching in the lower abdomen
   B. a painless lump on a testicle
   C. testicular swelling
   D. all of the above

_____ 2. Which of the following are known risk factors for testicular cancer?
   A. cryptorchidism
   B. a family history of testicular cancer
   C. both A and B
   D. none of the above

_____ 3. What is the single most important risk factor for prostate cancer?
   A. a family history of prostate cancer
   B. age
   C. smoking
   D. high-fat diet

Chapter 20

Practice Test

Completion: *Write the term that completes the statement in the space provided.*

1. _____ produces offspring that are identical to each other and to the parent.

2. Inherited genes are either _____ or recessive.

3. The _____ is lined with endometrial tissue, and houses and nurtures the developing fetus.

4. A girl's first menstrual cycle, or _____, typically occurs between 10 and 15 years of age.

5. _____ is the period of time between fertilization and birth.

True/False: *Indicate whether each statement below is true or false by circling either T or F.*

T   F   6. Semen is another name for sperm.

T   F   7. A fetus' lungs and heart are the last organs to complete development.

T   F   8. Prenatal care is provided after the baby is born.

T   F   9. Pregnant teens have high-risk pregnancies because their bodies have not finished maturing.

T   F   10. Pelvic inflammatory disease (PID) is a highly preventable condition.

Multiple Choice: *Write the letter that corresponds to the correct answer in the blank space.*

_____ 11. _____ is a condition in which a pregnant woman experiences high blood pressure.
   A. Gestational diabetes mellitus   C. Preeclampsia
   B. Hypertension   D. Ectopic pregnancy

_____ 12. Germ layers are embryonic tissues that will eventually constitute the _____ main types of tissues in the body.
   A. three   C. four
   B. two   D. five

_____ 13. In humans, sperm and ova are produced by a special type of cell division called _____.
   A. mitosis   C. sexual reproduction
   B. meiosis   D. fertilization

_____ 14. The _____ serves as the birth canal.
   A. uterus   C. vagina
   B. fallopian tubes   D. external genitalia

_____ 15. The _____ is a ball of cells formed by the cleaving zygote as it travels into the uterus.
   A. blastocyst   C. embryo
   B. chorion   D. placenta

Name _____ Date _____

Matching: *Match each key term to its definition by writing the letter of the term in the space provided.*

_____ 16. a condition in which an embryo implants and begins developing in the fallopian tubes

_____ 17. a long, whip-like structure on the sperm that propels the sperm through liquid

_____ 18. a pregnancy that ends before the twentieth week

_____ 19. spongy tissue that fills with blood during sexual excitement

_____ 20. a tube in the male reproductive system that carries sperm from the testes to the penis

_____ 21. the release of an ovum from one of the follicles in the ovaries

_____ 22. an organ filled with erectile tissue and located above the vaginal opening

B. miscarriage

C. flagellum

D. ectopic pregnancy

E. ovulation

F. clitoris

G. vas deferens

H. erectile tissue

Analyzing Data: *The graph below shows the birth rates for US women, ages 15–44, before and after the economic recession in 2008. Use the information provided to answer the following questions.*

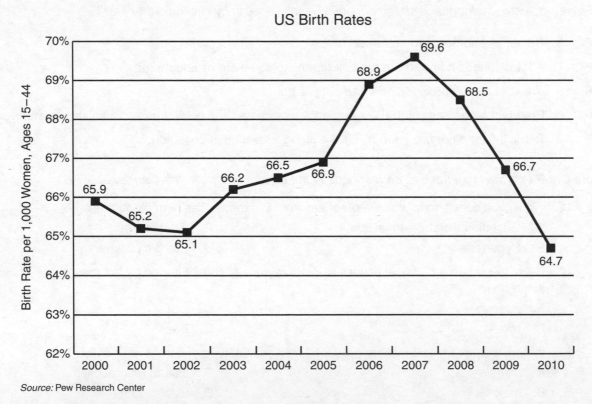

US Birth Rates

Source: Pew Research Center

23. For every 1,000 women, how many more babies were born in 2006 than in 2002?

_____

24. In which year were the fewest babies born?

_____

Short Answer: *On a separate sheet of paper, answer the following questions using what you have learned in this chapter.*

25. What is the difference between mitosis and meiosis?

26. Which five pregnancy complications are teens at an increased risk for developing?

Lesson 21.1

Key Terms Review

Multiple Choice: *Write the letter that corresponds to the correct answer in the blank space.*

_____ 1. The muscle contractions and changes that occur in a woman's body as she gives birth are known as _____.
A. dilation
B. epidural
C. reflexes
D. labor

_____ 2. The _____ test measures a newborn's health and condition through five basic tests.
A. oxytocin
B. Apgar
C. cesarean
D. vernix

_____ 3. A(n) _____ is an automatic muscle movement in response to a stimulus.
A. reflex
B. dilation
C. vernix
D. adoption

_____ 4. Which of the following terms describes an outline of a mother's preferences for the birth process?
A. birth plan
B. epidural
C. birthing room
D. episiotomy

_____ 5. A(n) _____ section is the delivery of an infant through an incision made in the mother's abdomen and uterus.
A. cesarean
B. vernix
C. Apgar
D. birthing

_____ 6. Which of the following is *not* a condition assessed by the Apgar test?
A. pulse
B. appearance
C. gender
D. respiration

_____ 7. A _____ is a private space, often within a hospital, where a mother can give birth surrounded by the familiar comforts of home.
A. private facility
B. birthing center
C. NICU
D. birthing room

(Continued)

_____ 8. The temporary, white protective coating that may cover a newborn at birth is known as _____.

    A. reflexes

    B. vernix

    C. dilation

    D. oxytocin

_____ 9. A certified _____ is a medical professional licensed to help women with routine, uncomplicated births.

    A. nurse-midwife

    B. adoption specialist

    C. OB/GYN

    D. labor coach

_____ 10. Which of the following is a hormone that triggers strong uterine contractions to push the baby through the cervix and vagina?

    A. dopamine

    B. estrogen

    C. testosterone

    D. oxytocin

_____ 11. A(n) _____ adoption occurs when an infant or child is adopted from another country or culture.

    A. open

    B. transcultural

    C. closed

    D. special

_____ 12. If a baby is having difficulty passing through the birth canal, a doctor may make an incision known as a(n) _____.

    A. episiotomy

    B. dilation

    C. vernix

    D. reflex

_____ 13. Which of the following is a nonmedical facility where a mother can give birth in a homelike environment?

    A. birthing plan

    B. birthing room

    C. birthing space

    D. birthing center

_____ 14. Which of the following is a pain medication used during childbirth?

    A. oxytocin

    B. vernix

    C. epidural anesthesia

    D. phenylketonuria

_____ 15. _____ describes the widening and thinning of the cervix.

    A. Dilation

    B. Vernix

    C. Reflex

    D. Birthing

Options for Childbirth

The process of childbirth is physically demanding and often painful. Making choices before childbirth can reduce stress in the moment, which is beneficial for both mother and baby. Listed below are a few of the choices a mother can make before childbirth. For each choice, research the options a mother has and use at least two online sources. Record your findings, and then express which option you think would be best for a mother and her baby.

Choice: What will be the birth setting?

Option #1: *birthing room*

Sources of information: _____

_____

Opinion: _____

_____

_____

Option #2: *birthing center*

_____

Sources of information: _____

Opinion: _____

_____

_____

Option #3: *at-home delivery*

Sources of information: _____

_____

Opinion: _____

_____

_____

Choice: Who will deliver the baby?

Option #1: *OB/GYN*

Sources of information: _____

_____

Opinion: _____

_____

_____

(Continued)

Name _____

Option #2: *family doctor*

Sources of information: _____

_____

Opinion: _____

_____

_____

Option #3: *nurse-midwife*

Sources of information: _____

_____

Opinion: _____

_____

_____

Choice: How will labor and delivery be managed?

Option #1: *epidural anesthesia*

Sources of information: _____

_____

Opinion: _____

_____

_____

_____

Option #2: *cesarean section*

Sources of information: _____

_____

Opinion: _____

_____

_____

_____

Lesson 21.2

Finding Reliable Health Information

For this activity, you will find three sources of reliable information for each of the three topics listed below. You may use the sources of information given in Figure 1.6, "Health and Safety Information," or you may research your own sources. For each source, write the name of the organization and the title of the article or web page. If the source does not appear in Figure 1.6, list its website address as well. Do not use a source more than once.

Topic: *Preventing sudden infant death syndrome (SIDS)*

1. A. Website #1 (name of organization) _____
   B. Title of article or web page _____
2. A. Website #2 (name of organization) _____
   B. Title of article or web page _____
3. A. Website #3 (name of organization) _____
   B. Title of article or web page _____

Topic: *Disposable diapers versus cloth diapers*

1. A. Website #1 (name of organization) _____
   B. Title of article or web page _____
2. A. Website #2 (name of organization) _____
   B. Title of article or web page _____
3. A. Website #3 (name of organization) _____
   B. Title of article or web page _____

Topic: *Immunizations for children*

1. A. Website #1 (name of organization) _____
   B. Title of article or web page _____
2. A. Website #2 (name of organization) _____
   B. Title of article or web page _____
3. A. Website #3 (name of organization) _____
   B. Title of article or web page _____

After compiling the above information about your sources, answer the following questions:

1. Of the three sources you chose for each topic, which sources were most reliable? How do you know?

   _____

   _____

2. Which sources provided the most interesting information? Write three facts you learned about each topic.

   _____

   _____

Name _____ Date _____

Breast-Feeding versus Formula-Feeding

While breast-feeding and formula-feeding will both meet an infant's nutritional needs, each of these methods has advantages and disadvantages. Read the lists below. One column gives facts about breast-feeding, and the other gives facts about formula-feeding. When you have read both lists, use the space at the bottom of this page to describe which method you think better meets a baby's nutritional needs. Also describe what factors might affect a mother's decision to breast-feed or formula-feed. Explain your answers clearly and use facts from the lists.

Breast-Feeding

- Immediately after a baby's birth, a mother's breasts make colostrum. Colostrum has more protein and antibodies than regular breast milk.

- Breast milk contains sugar, fat, protein, vitamins, minerals, and water in the right proportions for babies. Breast milk also contains antibodies to fight infection.

- Pediatricians recommend that breast milk be the only source of nutrition for the first six months of a baby's life.

- Breast-feeding is the natural form of nutrition for babies.

- Breast-feeding lowers babies' risks for developing diabetes, asthma, allergies, and obesity.

- Breast-feeding helps the mother lose weight, causes her uterus to return to normal, and may reduce her risk for breast or ovarian cancer.

- Breast-feeding is not an option for women who are taking medications for cancer or who have HIV/AIDS.

- Mothers may be unable to breast-feed due to work schedules.

- Breast-feeding costs very little.

- Breast-feeding is demanding for the mother.

- Breast milk can be pumped and stored in bottles for later.

Formula-Feeding

- Infant formula closely replicates the nutrients and caloric contents of breast milk.

- Formula-feeding allows mothers to share feeding responsibilities with the father and other family members.

- Babies digest formula more slowly than breast milk, which means they feed less often, allowing caretakers to rest.

- Formula-feeding allows mothers to monitor how much their babies are consuming.

- Formula-feeding is more expensive than breast-feeding.

- Formula-feeding requires more planning than breast-feeding.

- Caretakers must always have formula prepared and refrigerated with a steady supply of clean bottles.

- Formula-feeding does not typically cause conflicts with work schedules.

_____

_____

_____

_____

_____

_____

Name _____ Date _____

Lesson 21.5

Teen Parent Challenges

Teen parents face many challenges, including a lack of the time, energy, and financial resources that taking care of a new baby requires. Teens often have to drop out of school and find a job to earn more money. Understanding the challenges that teen parents face can help you understand the importance of thinking about the future when making choices today. For this activity, research each of the challenges of teen parenting listed below. Find at least two sources of reliable health information regarding these issues. List your findings and write a few sentences of reflection on what you have learned.

Challenge: Isolation from family and friends

Sources of information: _____
_____

Findings: _____
_____

Reflection: _____
_____
_____

Challenge: Financial strain

Sources of information: _____
_____

Findings: _____
_____

Reflection: _____
_____
_____

Challenge: Increased responsibilities

Sources of information: _____
_____

Findings: _____
_____

Reflection: _____
_____
_____

Name _____ Date _____

Infant Care Careers

In the Spotlight on Health and Wellness Careers feature in this chapter, several careers that relate to infant care are discussed. When choosing a career, you should be mindful of your personal interests, strengths, and weaknesses. These will help you decide which career would best suit you. Study the chart below, which is organized according to interest or personal quality, and then answer the questions that follow. Keep in mind your own interests, strengths, and weaknesses when reviewing the chart.

Interest/Quality	Career	Duties	Education and Training	Resources
Enjoys working with infants	Pediatric nurse	Delivers healthcare for newborns and infants	Associate's degree or bachelor's degree	American Nurses Association
	Certified nurse-midwife	Provides postnatal care	College degree, graduate training, certification	American College of Nurse-Midwives
	Obstetrician	Provides postnatal care	Bachelor's degree, medical degree	American Medical Association, American Congress of Obstetricians and Gynecologists
	Licensed practical nurse (LPN)	Administers basic nursing care to all patients	High school diploma, LPN certification/license	National Federation of Licensed Practical Nurses
Would enjoy assisting with childbirth	Certified nurse-midwife	Provides assistance with delivery	College degree, graduate training, certification	American College of Nurse-Midwives
	Obstetrician	Delivers babies	Bachelor's degree, medical degree	American Medical Association, American Congress of Obstetricians and Gynecologists
Is interested in science	Obstetrician	Diagnoses and treats conditions related to pregnancy and childbirth	Bachelor's degree, medical degree	American Medical Association, American Congress of Obstetricians and Gynecologists
Enjoys working with patients of all ages	Licensed practical nurse (LPN)	Administers basic nursing care	High school diploma, LPN certification/license	National Federation of Licensed Practical Nurses

1. Which of these careers lines up best with your interests or personality?

   _____

   _____

   _____

   _____

   _____

2. Choose one career to research further. For that career, visit the resource listed in the chart and compose a "day in the life" for someone with that career. Does this type of workday sound interesting to you?

   _____

   _____

   _____

   _____

   _____

3. According to the chart, which level of education is necessary for your chosen career? Research community colleges and universities in your area and plot out an educational plan to follow if you want this career.

   _____

   _____

   _____

   _____

   _____

4. Visit the *Occupational Outlook Handbook* online to research the job outlook for this particular career. Record your findings here.

   _____

   _____

   _____

   _____

5. According to the *Occupational Outlook Handbook*, what is a typical salary for someone in this career?

   _____

   _____

   _____

   _____

   _____

Chapter 21

Reading Practice

Reread the following passage from the textbook. Then answer the questions that follow.

Baby's First Medical Exam

After birth, a doctor assesses a newborn's general condition by using the *Apgar test*. This test is the acronym for the five conditions it assesses:

1. appearance (skin coloration)

2. pulse (heart rate)

3. grimace response (responsiveness to stimulation)

4. activity and muscle tone

5. respiration (breathing rate and effort)

The doctor rates each condition on a scale of 0 to 2, with 2 being the best. The scores for each condition are added to give the total Apgar score, which ranges from 10 (highest) to 0 (lowest). The Apgar test is usually given to a baby at one minute after birth and again at five minutes after birth. If the score at five minutes is low, the test may be administered for a third time at ten minutes after birth.

A score of eight after five minutes means the baby is in good health. Lower scores are common and usually mean the baby needs some attention or more time to adapt. When a very low score persists, something else may be wrong.

In addition to the Apgar test, a doctor does a physical exam and standard blood tests to detect any diseases or abnormalities. A tiny amount of blood is drawn from a heel prick to test for blood sugar abnormalities, thyroid disease, and *phenylketonuria (PKU)*, an inherited metabolic disease. These tests are done right away because these diseases can be controlled if detected early.

_____ 1. What is the main idea of this passage?

A. Respiration is important in determining a newborn's condition.

B. Phenylketonuria is an inherited metabolic disease.

C. The Apgar test is used to assess a newborn's general condition.

D. The Apgar test may be administered a third time ten minutes after birth.

_____ 2. One component measured by the Apgar test is *grimace response*, which is the baby's _____.

A. responsiveness to stimulation

B. muscle tone

C. breathing rate

D. skin coloration

_____ 3. In addition to the Apgar test, a doctor performs a _____ on the newborn.

A. reflex test

B. vernix assessment

C. dilation test

D. physical exam

_____ 4. The highest score a baby can receive on the Apgar test is _____.

A. 10

B. 8

C. 6

D. 7

Chapter 21

Practice Test

Completion: *Write the term that completes the statement in the space provided.*

1. Medical professionals known as_____ can assist women in uncomplicated births.

2. To prevent SIDS, babies should sleep on their _____.

3. During the first 30 days, infants can gain _____ ounce each day.

4. Soon after birth, babies and their parents or caregivers form an intimate, emotional connection known as a(n) _____.

5. _____ laws allow parents to leave their infants at designated locations if they wish to give up their infants for adoption.

True/False: *Indicate whether each statement below is true or false by circling either T or F.*

T   F   6. A medical process called *induction* can help speed up the delivery process.

T   F   7. Babies can be left alone on tables or in cribs with the side down.

T   F   8. Parents and caregivers should not respond to a baby's crying.

T   F   9. Most full-term babies triple their birth weight in one year.

T   F   10. Teen fathers have no responsibilities to their children.

Multiple Choice: *Write the letter that corresponds to the correct answer in the blank space.*

_____ 11. Regular contractions of the uterus cause the cervix to _____ and _____.
   A. open, close
   B. push, pull
   C. thin, stretch
   D. contract, expand

_____ 12. Which of the following diseases can be prevented by a vaccine?
   A. whooping cough
   B. diaper rash
   C. SIDS
   D. fever

_____ 13. Which of the following statements is true of breast-feeding?
   A. Breast-feeding has no advantages for the mother.
   B. Breast milk does not help babies fight infections.
   C. Breast milk is the natural form of nutrition for babies.
   D. All women can breast-feed.

_____ 14. Babies may cry when they are _____.
   A. hungry
   B. sleepy
   C. stressed
   D. all of the above

_____ 15. Which of the following are major expenses for teen parents?
   A. education
   B. healthcare
   C. child care
   D. all of the above

(Continued)

Matching: *Match each key term to its definition by writing the letter of the term in the space provided.*

_____ 16. an automatic muscle movement in which an infant turns his or her head and tries to suck when hungry

_____ 17. the death of a healthy baby while sleeping

_____ 18. a healthcare professional who counsels and assists new mothers as they breast-feed their babies

_____ 19. the financial contribution legally required of a noncustodial parent

_____ 20. a protein- and antibody-rich substance secreted from a mother's breasts for a few days after she gives birth

_____ 21. trauma and brain damage caused by an infant being jostled or handled roughly

_____ 22. a parent who does not provide primary care for a child, but has legal rights and responsibilities regarding the child

A. child support

B. colostrum

C. lactation consultant

D. noncustodial parent

E. rooting reflex

F. shaken baby syndrome

G. sudden infant death syndrome (SIDS)

Analyzing Data: *The graph below compares the levels of education achieved by teens who have given birth and the levels of education achieved by teens who have not given birth. Study the data in this graph and then answer the questions that follow.*

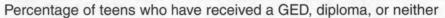

Percentage of teens who have received a GED, diploma, or neither

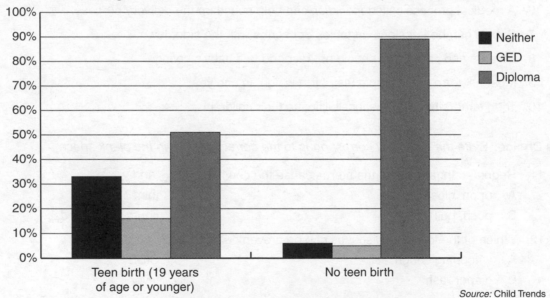

Source: Child Trends

23. What percentage of teens who gave birth achieved neither a GED nor a diploma?

_____

24. What is the ratio of teens who have not given birth and attained a diploma to teens who *have* given birth and attained a diploma?

_____

Short Answer: *On a separate sheet of paper, answer the following questions using what you have learned in this chapter.*

25. What are some pros and cons of disposable and cloth diapers? Which type of diaper do you think is the better choice?

26. Given what you have learned about caring for newborns, why might parents be frustrated during the first few months of parenthood?

Lesson 22.1

The Human Life Cycle

The human life cycle consists of several developmental stages, each of which lasts for a set amount of time and contains its own well-known important events, or milestones. Milestones can include walking, going to school, learning to drive, or getting married. For each of the developmental stages listed below, identify the age range associated with that stage and list one or two milestones you think might correspond to that stage. When you have finished, compare responses with your classmates.

Stage: Infancy

Age range: _____

Milestones: _____

_____

Stage: Toddlerhood

Age range: _____

Milestones: _____

_____

Stage: Preschool

Age range: _____

Milestones: _____

_____

Stage: School-age

Age range: _____

Milestones: _____

_____

Stage: Adolescence

Age range: _____

Milestones: _____

_____

Stage: Adulthood

Age range: _____

Milestones: _____

_____

Lesson 22.1

Your Life Span, Your Choices

Life span is the number of years an individual actually lives. Each person's life span depends on his or her genes, environment, and lifestyle. Making unhealthy life choices can cause your physical health and appearance to decline as you age. Making healthy life choices can make aging easier. Consider each of the lifestyle choices listed here and determine whether each choice is healthy or unhealthy. Then, list ways in which a person might benefit from or suffer as a result of these choices.

1. **Choice: Smoking for many years**

   A. Is this choice healthy or unhealthy?_____

   B. What are the consequences or benefits of this choice?

   _____

   _____

2. **Choice: Maintaining good nutrition**

   A. Is this choice healthy or unhealthy?_____

   B. What are the consequences or benefits of this choice?

   _____

   _____

3. **Choice: Sitting down most of the day**

   A. Is this choice healthy or unhealthy?_____

   B. What are the consequences or benefits of this choice?

   _____

   _____

4. **Choice: Quitting smoking**

   A. Is this choice healthy or unhealthy?_____

   B. What are the consequences or benefits of this choice?

   _____

   _____

5. **Choice: Eating lots of junk food**

   A. Is this choice healthy or unhealthy?_____

   B. What are the consequences or benefits of this choice?

   _____

   _____

6. **Choice: Being physically active**

   A. Is this choice healthy or unhealthy?_____

   B. What are the consequences or benefits of this choice?

   _____

   _____

Infancy through Preschool Years

The first five years of a person's life are marked by important milestones that develop a person's most basic functions. Infants learn to walk and become toddlers who are constantly on the move. Toddlers grow into curious preschoolers. During early childhood, growth and development are achieved in four areas—physical development, intellectual development, emotional development, and social development. For each of the scenarios below, identify the individual's stage of life (infancy, toddlerhood, or preschool), and identify what type of developmental milestone is taking place.

1. Joey learns how to feed himself by holding a cup and spoon on his own.

   A. What is Joey's stage of life? _____

   B. In what developmental area does this milestone fall? Explain your answer.

   _____

2. Casey realizes that shaking her rattle causes it to make a noise.

   A. What is Casey's stage of life? _____

   B. In what developmental area does this milestone fall? Explain your answer.

   _____

3. Bradley watches other children play in the park and enjoys playing on his own near them.

   A. What is Bradley's stage of life? _____

   B. In what developmental area does this milestone fall? Explain your answer.

   _____

4. Baby Kate forms a strong, emotional connection to her mother as her mother talks and laughs with her.

   A. What is Kate's stage of life?_____

   B. In what developmental area does this milestone fall? Explain your answer.

   _____

5. Gerry uses child safety scissors to cut up colorful paper.

   A. What is Gerry's stage of life?_____

   B. In what developmental area does this milestone fall? Explain your answer.

   _____

6. Darla imitates the way her mother always says, "oh my goodness!"

   A. What is Darla's stage of life? _____

   B. In what developmental area does this milestone fall? Explain your answer.

   _____

Lesson 22.2

Key Terms Review

Multiple Choice: *Write the letter that corresponds to the correct answer in the blank space.*

_____ 1. _____ skills involve movements that use the body's small muscles.
   A. Walking   C. Physical
   B. Fine-motor   D. Gross-motor

_____ 2. A child's fear of unfamiliar people or situations is known as _____.
   A. stranger anxiety   C. separation anxiety
   B. attachment anxiety   D. autonomy

_____ 3. _____ is the idea that objects and people are present even when they cannot be seen.
   A. Stranger anxiety   C. Separation anxiety
   B. Attachment   D. Object permanence

_____ 4. _____ development involves the increase in a person's coordination and strength of muscles.
   A. Motor   C. Social
   B. Intellectual   D. Physical

_____ 5. The freedom to direct one's self independent of other influences is known as _____.
   A. reception   C. autonomy
   B. motor skills   D. attachment

_____ 6. _____ skills involve movements that use the large muscles of the body.
   A. Attachment   C. Intellectual
   B. Fine-motor   D. Gross-motor

_____ 7. Which of the following terms describes a frustrated or angry reaction that includes crying, yelling, or mild physical violence?
   A. autonomy   C. stranger anxiety
   B. temper tantrum   D. empathy

_____ 8. _____ play occurs when preschoolers play with other children.
   A. Parallel   C. Cooperative
   B. Tantrum   D. Attachment

_____ 9. A child's fear of being away from his or her caregiver is called _____.
   A. separation anxiety   C. stranger anxiety
   B. attachment anxiety   D. temper tantrum

_____ 10. The term _____ describes an emotional connection, especially between a baby and his or her caregiver.
   A. *autonomy*   C. *permanence*
   B. *development*   D. *attachment*

Name _____ Date _____

Finding Reliable Health Information

For this activity, you will find three sources of reliable information for each of the three topics listed below. You may use the sources of information given in Figure 1.6, "Health and Safety Information," or you may research your own sources. For each source, write the name of the organization and the title of the article or web page. If the source does not appear in Figure 1.6, list its website address as well. Do not use a source more than once.

Topic: *Adolescent health and wellness*

1. A. Website #1 (name of organization) _____

   B. Title of article or web page _____

2. A. Website #2 (name of organization) _____

   B. Title of article or web page _____

3. A. Website #3 (name of organization) _____

   B. Title of article or web page _____

Topic: *Adolescent brain development*

1. A. Website #1 (name of organization) _____

   B. Title of article or web page _____

2. A. Website #2 (name of organization) _____

   B. Title of article or web page _____

3. A. Website #3 (name of organization) _____

   B. Title of article or web page _____

Topic: *Adolescents and independence*

1. A. Website #1 (name of organization) _____

   B. Title of article or web page _____

2. A. Website #2 (name of organization) _____

   B. Title of article or web page _____

3. A. Website #3 (name of organization) _____

   B. Title of article or web page _____

After compiling the above information about your sources, answer the following questions:

1. Of the three sources you chose for each topic, which sources were most reliable? How do you know?

_____

_____

2. Which sources provided the most interesting information? Write three facts you learned about each topic.

_____

_____

Lesson 22.4

Understanding Adulthood

In the United States, people are generally considered to be adults when they reach 18 years of age. At this time, a person can vote, get married, and be tried as an adult in court. However, after 18 years of age, adults continue to change and develop through various stages of adulthood. Interview someone you know who fits into each of the stages of adulthood—young adulthood, middle age, and older adulthood. Ask your interviewee each of the questions provided, and ask at least one other question that you want answered. Record the answers here.

Young Adulthood

Name of interviewee:_____

Questions

1. Since there is no "typical" young adult in the United States, what is your definition of young adulthood?

   _____
   _____
   _____
   _____

2. What has been the biggest change in your life from adolescence to young adulthood?

   _____
   _____
   _____
   _____

3. (Your question)_____

   (Answer)_____
   _____
   _____
   _____

Middle Age

Name of interviewee:_____

Questions

1. Were you worried about entering middle age? Were those worries valid?

   _____
   _____
   _____
   _____

Name _____

2. What has surprised you the most about middle age?

_____

_____

_____

_____

_____

3. (Your question)_____

(Answer)_____

_____

_____

_____

_____

_____

Older Adulthood

Name of interviewee:_____

Questions

1. What do you spend most of your time doing?

_____

_____

_____

_____

_____

2. What is the greatest source of happiness in your life at this time?

_____

_____

_____

_____

_____

_____

3. (Your question)_____

(Answer)_____

_____

_____

_____

_____

Lesson 22.5

Older Adult Care Careers

In the Spotlight on Health and Wellness Careers feature in this chapter, several careers that relate to older adult care are discussed. When choosing a career, you should be mindful of your personal interests, strengths, and weaknesses. These will help you decide which career would best suit you. Study the chart below, which is organized according to interest or personal quality, and then answer the questions that follow. Keep in mind your own interests, strengths, and weaknesses when reviewing the chart.

Interest/Quality	Career	Duties	Education and Training	Resources
Good communication and listening skills	Recreational therapist	Directs recreational activities for older adults	Bachelor's degree and certification	American Therapeutic Recreation Association
	Geriatric social worker	Helps older adults solve problems	Master's degree	National Association of Social Workers
Enjoys working in a hospital setting	Nursing assistant or orderly	Works in hospitals or nursing homes	State-approved education program and competency exam, on-the-job training	National Association of Health Care Assistants
Wants to assist with social and emotional issues	Geriatric social worker	Helps older adults obtain medical, psychological, and financial assistance	Master's degree	National Association of Social Workers
	Rehabilitation counselor	Assists older adults with emotional problems associated with recovery from disabilities and diseases	Master's degree and state license	American Rehabilitation Counseling Association
Wants to assist with physical issues	Recreational therapist	Plans, directs, and coordinates recreational activities	Bachelor's degree and certification	American Therapeutic Recreation Association
	Nursing assistant or orderly	Provides basic care and assistance for activities of daily living	State-approved education program and competency exam, on-the-job training	National Association of Health Care Assistants
	Rehabilitation counselor	Assists older adults with physical problems associated with recovery from disabilities and diseases	Master's degree and state license	American Rehabilitation Counseling Association

Name _____

1. Which of these careers lines up best with your interests or personality?

_____

_____

_____

_____

2. Choose one career to research further. For that career, visit the resource listed in the chart and compose a "day in the life" for someone with that career. Does this type of workday sound interesting to you?

_____

_____

_____

_____

_____

3. According to the chart, which level of education is necessary for your chosen career? Research community colleges and universities in your area and plot out an educational plan to follow if you want this career.

_____

_____

_____

_____

_____

4. Visit the *Occupational Outlook Handbook* online to research the job outlook for this particular career. Record your findings here.

_____

_____

_____

_____

5. According to the *Occupational Outlook Handbook*, what is a typical salary for someone in this career?

_____

_____

_____

_____

_____

Chapter 22

Reading Practice

Reread the following passage from the textbook. Then answer the questions that follow.

Interactions with Caregivers

Around one year of age, children may become upset, shy, or afraid around unfamiliar people and in new situations. This is a normal developmental milestone called **stranger anxiety**. Caregivers can help children with stranger anxiety by gradually and patiently introducing them to new people and places.

Young children may also develop **separation anxiety**, meaning they become upset when they are away from their caregivers. Without a good understanding of time, children do not know how long these important people will be gone. Separation anxiety is normal and usually stops when a child is between two and three years of age.

The phrase *terrible twos* is often used to describe toddlers' behavior between two and three years of age. This age is characterized by the toddler alternating between displays of **autonomy** (self-directing freedom) and independence, and clinging, dependent behavior. Toddlers often react with frustration and anger—including yelling, crying, hitting, biting, or kicking—when they are prevented from doing what they want. This is called a **temper tantrum**. These reactions are normal and are simply the way toddlers test limits. Caregivers need to define limits and teach toddlers which behaviors (hitting, for example) are unacceptable. Toddlers will eventually learn these limits.

_____ 1. Which of the following is true of stranger anxiety?

A. Stranger anxiety is not normal and should concern parents.

B. Stranger anxiety signals delayed social development.

C. Stranger anxiety is a normal developmental milestone.

D. Stranger anxiety is typical of newborns.

_____ 2. _____ is normal and usually stops when a child is between two and three years of age.

A. Attachment

B. Empathy

C. Caregiving

D. Separation anxiety

_____ 3. Which of the following is *not* included in a temper tantrum?

A. kicking

B. hitting

C. hugging

D. biting

_____ 4. _____ is a sense of how another person may be feeling.

A. Attachment

B. Autonomy

C. Anxiety

D. Empathy

Chapter 22

Practice Test

Completion: *Write the term that completes the statement in the space provided.*

1. The quality of one person or piece of information being reliant on another is called
   _____.

2. By the preschool years, children develop keen _____ skills, which enable
   them to sort toys and other objects.

3. During the school-age years, children develop their _____, which is their
   sense of worth, purpose, security, and confidence.

4. The term _____ describes adults who care for their parents as well as their
   children.

5. The goal of _____ is to bring comfort and pain relief to patients who are being
   treated for diseases or disorders.

True/False: *Indicate whether each statement below is true or false by circling either T or F.*

T   F   6. Some people reach developmental milestones earlier or later than their peers.

T   F   7. Toddlers engage in cooperative play rather than parallel play.

T   F   8. In females, puberty begins between 10 and 16 years of age.

T   F   9. Older adults have to deal with body system changes, such as incontinence.

T   F   10. Not all people experience the acceptance stage of grief.

Multiple Choice: *Write the letter that corresponds to the correct answer in the blank space.*

_____ 11. Which of the following is *not* a developmental stage in the human life cycle?
   A. adulthood   C. toddlerhood
   B. puberty   D. school-age

_____ 12. As they improve their _____, children develop precise, refined muscle movements and
   coordination.
   A. gross-motor skills   C. receptive language
   B. classification skills   D. pincer grasp

_____ 13. Puberty begins in males with enlargement of the _____.
   A. testes   C. shoulders
   B. stomach   D. muscles

_____ 14. Which of the following life stages is also known as *middle age*?
   A. sandwich generation   C. young adulthood
   B. middle adulthood   D. older adulthood

_____ 15. The _____ stage of grief includes deep sadness.
   A. bargaining   C. denial
   B. anger   D. depression

(Continued)

Name _____ Date _____

Matching: *Match each key term to its definition by writing the letter of the term in the space provided.*

_____ 16. the sequence of developmental stages in a person's life span

_____ 17. ejaculations of semen while sleeping

_____ 18. an arrangement outlining how possessions, land, and property are to be divided upon a person's death

_____ 19. the period during which levels of sex hormones increase and primary and secondary sexual characteristics develop

_____ 20. healthcare designed to provide comfort for terminally ill patients and their families

_____ 21. the inability to prevent urination when urine accumulates in the bladder

_____ 22. a condition of mental deterioration

A. dementia

B. hospice care

C. human life cycle

D. incontinence

E. last will and testament

F. nocturnal emissions

G. puberty

Analyzing Data: *The graph below illustrates the effects of body weight and physical activity on life expectancy. Study the data in this graph and then answer the questions that follow.*

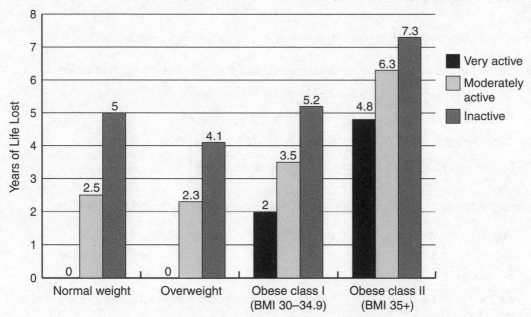

Effect of Body Weight and Physical Activity on Life Expectancy

23. In the overweight category, what is the difference in years of life lost between a moderately active person and an inactive person?

_____

24. How many more years of life does a moderately active person in *obese class* I lose in comparison to a moderately active overweight person?

_____

Short Answer: *On a separate sheet of paper, answer the following questions using what you have learned in this chapter.*

25. What do you think is the definition of adulthood in the United States today? Explain your answer.

26. Explain the importance of a durable power of attorney for healthcare.

Notes

Notes